Lecture Notes in Computer Science 11851

More information about this series at http://www.springer.com/series/7412

Luping Zhou · Nicholas Heller ·
Yiyu Shi · Yiming Xiao et al. (Eds.)

Large-Scale Annotation of Biomedical Data and Expert Label Synthesis and Hardware Aware Learning for Medical Imaging and Computer Assisted Intervention

International Workshops, LABELS 2019,
HAL-MICCAI 2019, and CuRIOUS 2019
Held in Conjunction with MICCAI 2019
Shenzhen, China, October 13 and 17, 2019
Proceedings

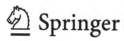 Springer

Editors
Luping Zhou
University of Sydney
Sydney, NSW, Australia

Nicholas Heller
University of Minnesota
Minneapolis, MN, USA

Yiyu Shi
University of Notre Dame
Notre Dame, IN, USA

Yiming Xiao 🅳
Western University
London, ON, Canada

Additional Workshop Editors *see next page*

ISSN 0302-9743   ISSN 1611-3349   (electronic)
Lecture Notes in Computer Science
ISBN 978-3-030-33641-7   ISBN 978-3-030-33642-4   (eBook)
https://doi.org/10.1007/978-3-030-33642-4

LNCS Sublibrary: SL6 – Image Processing, Computer Vision, Pattern Recognition, and Graphics

This Springer imprint is published by the registered company Springer Nature Switzerland AG
The registered company address is: Gewerbestrasse 11, 6330 Cham, Switzerland

Additional Workshop Editors

Satellite Events Chair

Kenji Suzuki
Tokyo Institute of Technology
Yokohama, Japan

Workshop Chairs

Hongen Liao
Tsinghua University
Beijing, China

Hayit Greenspan
Tel Aviv University
Tel Aviv, Israel

Challenge Chairs

Qian Wang
Shanghai Jiaotong University
Shanghai, China

Bram van Ginneken
Radboud University
Nijmegen, The Netherlands

Tutorial Chair

Luping Zhou
University of Sydney
Sydney, Australia

LABELS 2019 Editors

Nicholas Heller
University of Minnesota
Minneapolis, MN, USA

Diana Mateus
École Centrale de Nantes
Nantes, France

Raphael Sznitman
University of Bern
Bern, Switzerland

Emanuele Trucco
University of Dundee
Dundee, UK

Veronika Cheplygina
Eindhoven University of Technology
Eindhoven, The Netherlands

HAL-MICCAI 2019 Editors

Yiyu Shi
University of Notre Dame
Notre Dame, IN, USA

Danny Chen
University of Notre Dame
Notre Dame, IN, USA

X. Sharon Hu
University of Notre Dame
Notre Dame, IN, USA

CuRIOUS 2019 Editors

Yiming Xiao ⓘ
Western University
London, ON, Canada

Hassan Rivaz ⓘ
Concordia University
Montréal, QC, Canada

Matthieu Chabanas ⓘ
University of Grenoble Alpes
Grenoble, France

Ingerid Reinertsen ⓘ
Health Research
SINTEF Digital
Trondheim, Norway

LABELS 2019 Preface

This volume contains the proceedings of the 4th International Workshop on Large-scale Annotation of Biomedical data and Expert Label Synthesis (LABELS 2019), which was held on October 13, 2019, in conjunction with the 22nd International Conference on Medical Image Computing and Computer Assisted Intervention (MICCAI 2019) in Shenzhen, China. The first workshop in the LABELS series was held in 2016 in Athens, Greece. This was followed by workshops in Quebec City, Canada in 2017, and Granada, Spain in 2018.

With the widespread use of data-intensive supervised machine learning methods in medical image computing, a growing pressure has mounted to generate vast quantities of quality annotations. Unsurprisingly, in response to the need for very large volumes of training data for deep learning systems, the demand for new methods of gathering vast amounts of annotations in efficient, coherent, and safe ways has only grown. To address these issues, LABELS gathers contributions and approaches focused on either adapting supervised learning methods to learn from external types of labels (e.g., multiple instance learning, transfer learning) and/or acquiring more, or more informative, annotations, and thus reducing annotation costs (e.g., active learning, crowdsourcing). Following the success of the previous three LABELS workshops, and given the ever-growing need for such methods, the fourth workshop was planned for 2019. The workshop included invited talks by Annika Reinke (German Cancer Research Center, Germany) and Bjoern Menze (Technical University of Munich, Germany), as well as several papers and abstracts. After peer review, a total of eight papers and two abstracts were selected. The papers appear in this volume, and the abstracts are available on the workshop website: http://miccailabels.org. A variety of approaches for dealing with a limited number of labels, from semi-supervised learning to crowdsourcing, are well-represented within the workshop. Unlike many workshops, the contributions also feature "insightfully unsuccessful" results, which illustrate the difficulty of collecting annotations in the real world. We would like to thank all the speakers and authors for joining our workshop, the Program Committee for their excellent work with the peer reviews, our sponsors – RetinAi Medical and Auris Health – for their support, and the workshop chairs for their help with the organization of the fourth LABELS workshop.

September 2019

Nicholas Heller
Raphael Sznitman
Veronika Cheplygina
Diana Mateus
Emanuele Trucco

Organization

Organizing Committee

Nicholas Heller	University of Minnesota, USA
Raphael Sznitman	University of Bern, Switzerland
Veronika Cheplygina	Eindhoven University of Technology, The Netherlands
Diana Mateus	Technical University of Munich, Germany
Emanuele Trucco	University of Dundee, UK

Program Committee

Florian Dubost	Erasmus University MC, The Netherlands
Amelia Jimenez-Sanchez	Pompeu Fabra University, Spain
Obioma Pelka	University of Duisburg-Essen, Germany
Christoph Friedrich	University of Applied Sciences and Arts Dortmund, Germany
John Onofrey	Yale University, USA
Ke Yan	National Institutes of Health, USA
Vinkle Srivastav	University of Strasbourg, France
Loic Peter	University College London, UK
Jaime Cardoso	Universidade do Porto, Portugal
Filipe Condessa	Carnegie Mellon University, USA
Jack Rickman	University of Minnesota, USA
Bjoern Menze	Technical University of Munich, Germany
Roger Tam	University of British Columbia, Canada
Weidong Cai	University of Sydney, Australia
Silas Ørting	University of Copenhagen, Denmark
Joseph Jacobs	University College London, UK
Joshua Dean	University of Minnesota, USA

HAL-MICCAI 2019 Preface

With the prevalence of deep neural networks, machine intelligence has recently demonstrated performance comparable with, and in some cases superior to, that of human experts in medical imaging and computer assisted intervention. Such accomplishments can be largely credited to the ever-increasing computing power, as well as a growing abundance of medical data. As larger clusters of faster computing nodes become available at lower cost and in smaller form factors, more data can be used to train deeper neural networks with more layers and neurons, which usually translate to higher performance and at the same time higher computational complexity. For example, the widely used $3D$ U-Net for medical image segmentation has more than 16 million parameters and needs about 4.7×1013 floating point operations to process a $512 \times 512 \times 200$ $3D$ image. The large sizes and high computation complexity of neural networks have brought about two emerging issues that need to be addressed by the joint efforts between hardware designers and researchers in the MICCAI society towards hardware aware learning.

First, when powerful computing resources are easily accessible through network connection, such large networks may not impose significant challenges. However, for many medical applications where latency, privacy, or reliability is critical (such as implantable medical devices or health monitoring), inference has to be done locally, and such computation is subject to stringent area and power constraints due to limited resources available. To address the computational demands, hardware designers have started to explore techniques to compress deep neural networks for efficient local inference (i.e., edge inference). The ultimate judgment of such techniques is that lower power and area overhead can be achieved with minimal loss in inference accuracy. As many researchers in the MICCAI society are focusing on increasing inference accuracy through designing more complex networks, a correlated race exists between these researchers and hardware designers. Semiconductor technology scaling based on Moore's law has provided hardware designers a relatively easy path towards accommodating increasing network sizes. However, with the slowdown of the scaling trends, a clear gap between hardware capacity and computational demand has emerged. It would therefore be of interest to explore various hardware designs coupled with algorithm innovations that could help to bridge the gaps.

Second, in many real-time medical applications such as image/VR guided surgery, it is desirable to further accelerate the inference speed of large neural networks. As hardware acceleration of deep neural networks is popular today, it would be interesting to explore customized hardware that utilizes the dedicated structure of a network for maximal efficiency. On the other hand, for a given hardware platform, it would also be interesting to see how to design a neural network/algorithm that can work best with it for a particular medical application. Ultimately, the joint exploration/co-design of hardware and neural networks can benefit many important problems within the MICCAI scope.

The HAL-MICCAI 2019 proceedings contain five high-quality papers that were preselected through a rigorous peer-review process. All submissions were peer-reviewed through a double-blind process by at least 3 members of the Program Committee, comprising 11 experts in the field of hardware aware medical applications. The accepted manuscripts cover a wide set of hardware applications in medical problems, including medical image segmentation, electron tomography, pneumonia detection, etc. In addition to the papers presented in this LNCS volume, the workshop comprised a keynote speech from a world renowned expert Prof. Danny Chen on deep learning and medical image applications, and an invited talk from Prof. Cheng Zhuo on pathology image processing.

October 2019   Yiyu Shi
                                                             X. Sharon Hu
                                                              Danny Chen

Organization

Organizing Committee

Program Committee Chair

Yiyu Shi   University of Notre Dame, USA

Program Committee Co-chairs

X. Sharon Hu   University of Notre Dame, USA
Danny Chen   University of Notre Dame, USA

Publicity Chair

Bei Yu   Chinese University of Hong Kong, Hong Kong, China

Program Committee Members

Albert Liu   Kneron, USA
An Zeng   South China University of Technology, China
Guojie Luo   Peking University, China
Jian Zhuang   Guangdong General Hospital, China
Jianxu Chen   Allen Institute, USA
Jinjun Xiong   IBM T. J. Watson Research Center, USA
Lichuan Ping   Max BioE, USA
Steve Jiang   University of Texas Southwestern Medical Center, USA
Umamaheswara Rao Tida   North Dakota State University, USA
Yongpan Liu   Tsinghua University, China
Yu Wang   Tsinghua University, China

CuRIOUS 2019 Preface

Early brain tumor resection can effectively improve the patient's survival rate. However, resection quality and safety can often be heavily affected by intra-operative brain tissue shift due to factors, such as gravity, drug administration, intracranial pressure change, and tissue removal. Such tissue shift can displace the surgical target and vital structures (e.g., blood vessels) shown in pre-operative images while these displacements may not be directly visible in the surgeon's field of view. Intra-operative ultrasound (iUS) is a robust and relatively inexpensive technique to track intra-operative tissue shift and surgical tools. However, to help update pre-surgical plans with this information, accurate and robust image registration algorithms are needed to relate pre-surgical magnetic resonance imaging (MRI) scans to iUS images at different stages of the surgery. Despite the great progress so far, medical image registration techniques still have not made into the surgical room to directly benefit the patients with brain tumors. This second edition of the CuRIOUS MICCAI challenge provided a snapshot of the current progress in the field through extended discussions and provided researchers with an opportunity and common benchmark to characterize their inter-modal (MRI vs. iUS) and intra-modal image (iUS vs. iUS) registration methods on standardized datasets of iUS-guided brain tumor resection.

October 2019

Yiming Xiao
Matthieu Chabanas
Hassan Rivaz
Ingerid Reinertsen

Organization

Organization Committee

Yiming Xiao   Western University, Canada
Matthieu Chabanas   University of Grenoble Alpes, Grenoble, France
Hassan Rivaz   Concordia University, Canada
Ingerid Reinertsen   SINTEF, Norway

Contents

4th International Workshop on Large-Scale Annotation of Biomedical Data and Expert Label Synthesis (LABELS 2019)

Comparison of Active Learning Strategies Applied to Lung Nodule Segmentation in CT Scans

Daria Zotova[1,2], Aneta Lisowska[1(✉)], Owen Anderson[1,3], Vismantas Dilys[1], and Alison O'Neil[1,4]

[1] Canon Medical Research Europe, Edinburgh, UK
`aneta.lisowska@eu.medical.canon`
[2] Universitat de Girona, Girona, Spain
[3] University of Glasgow, Glasgow, UK
[4] University of Edinburgh, Edinburgh, UK

Abstract. Supervised machine learning techniques require large amounts of annotated training data to attain good performance. Active learning aims to ease the data collection process by automatically detecting which instances an expert should annotate in order to train a model as quickly and effectively as possible. Such strategies have been previously reported for medical imaging, but for other tasks than focal pathologies where there is high class imbalance and heterogeneous background appearance. In this study we evaluate different data selection approaches (random, uncertain, and representative sampling) and a semi-supervised model training procedure (pseudo-labelling), in the context of lung nodule segmentation in CT volumes from the publicly available LIDC-IDRI dataset. We find that active learning strategies allow us to train a model with equal performance but less than half of the annotation effort; data selection by uncertainty sampling offers the most gain, with the incorporation of representativeness or the addition of pseudo-labelling giving further small improvements. We conclude that active learning is a valuable tool and that further development of these strategies can play a key role in making diagnostic algorithms viable.

Keywords: Active learning · Lung nodule segmentation · Pseudo-labelling

1 Introduction

Data hungry deep learning techniques have become the 'go to' approach when it comes to pathology and organ segmentation in medical images, resulting in a high demand for annotated data. Usually annotation can only be performed by medical domain experts who have limited time to give, thus there is an interest in approaches which can reduce the annotation burden. Active learning

D. Zotova and A. Lisowska—Equal contribution

© Springer Nature Switzerland AG 2019
L. Zhou et al. (Eds.): LABELS 2019/HAL-MICCAI 2019/CuRIOUS 2019, LNCS 11851, pp. 3–12, 2019.
https://doi.org/10.1007/978-3-030-33642-4_1

techniques tackle this by putting the domain expert in the model training loop, and iteratively selecting subsets of unlabelled instances to annotate in order to induce the biggest boost in model performance [22]. In recent years there have been various active learning approaches proposed and applied to the tasks of melanoma segmentation in optical images [7], gland segmentation in histological images [22] and lymph node segmentation in ultrasound [22]. In this study we are interested in their performance in the setting of high class imbalance and heterogeneous background appearance, as is commonly the case for computer-aided diagnosis (CAD) tasks with focal pathologies.

Lung cancer is the second most common type of cancer diagnosed in the United States and the United Kingdom for both men and women [17], and screening with Computed Tomography (CT) scans is an effective tool for early diagnosis [1,4]. Consequently, creation of a robust system that detects lung nodules is one of the most commonly attempted medical image analysis tasks [6,8,11]. The contribution of this paper is a comparison of existing active learning approaches and analysis of their performance for lung nodule segmentation.

2   Related Work

Uncertainty sampling is a simple active learning strategy popularly used with various types of classifier [18]. In neural networks, uncertainty can be estimated by incorporating a dropout layer activated at inference time [5]. Gorriz *et al.* used this method in the context of melanoma segmentation [7], to obtain pixel-wise uncertainty maps for selection of the most *uncertain* samples for annotation. Further, building on previous work in image classification by Wang *et al.* [21], they used the uncertainty estimation to select the most *certain* samples and used the predictions as pseudo-labels for training. Pseudo-labelling is not novel; for instance, in [12] for image classification, the pseudo-label was defined simply as the class with the highest probability, while in [3] several techniques to obtain the confidence measure of pseudo-labels were proposed.

Yang *et al.* introduced a deep active learning framework that combines uncertainty sampling with representativeness estimation [22]. The representativeness measure was intended to select a set of samples which is representative of the variation in the unlabelled pool. Representativeness was measured by the mean cosine similarity between each sample in the unlabelled pool and its closest match in the candidate set, where matching was performed between the compressed representations learned by the network.

3   Methods

3.1   Data

We used CT scans from the publicly available Lung Image Database Consortium and Image Database Resource Initiative (LIDC-IDRI) collection [2]. The database consists of 1018 cases, each labelled with the nodule segmentations and the estimated malignancy (based on the image). In this study, a subset of 363 patients was used: 262 training (2973 nodules), 81 validation (991 nodules) and 20 test (239 nodules). We extracted the slices with nodules annotated by at least one annotator. Where there were multiple annotators per nodule, the union of the annotations was selected as the nodule mask. From each patient we also extracted a single random slice without nodules. This reduced dataset (i.e., subset of slices chosen for each patient) was pragmatically chosen to keep run times reasonable, since each active learning experiment run is itself the sum of many training runs. Images were pre-processed by clamping the pixel intensity values at −880 and 430 Hounsfield Units and rescaling to lie between 0 and 1.

3.2   Network Architecture and Parameters

We employed a 2D (slice-wise) VGG U-Net [16,19], constructed by using VGGNet as the encoder part of the U-Net and mirroring this with a similar decoder architecture, as shown in Fig. 1. There are three input channels to encode 3-D context information; we input the centre slice that contains the nodule and its neighbouring slices. The network was trained using a focal loss function [13] and the Adam optimiser [10] with a cyclical learning rate [20] and batches of 16 slices. Training was run for 200 epochs, with early stopping (patience of 20 epochs) and the best network weights on the validation set were retained according to a binary cross-entropy loss function (more stable than focal loss).

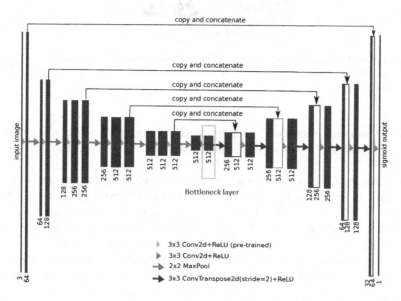

Fig. 1. Diagram of VGG U-Net. The bottleneck layer is marked in red: this is where uncertainty dropout is applied and where the compressed representation is derived. (Color figure online)

3.3   Active Learning Strategies

Our active learning setup is illustrated in Fig. 2. We implemented three active learning strategies as described below. Each strategy aims to select suitable annotated patients to add to the labelled set (in lieu of live annotation).

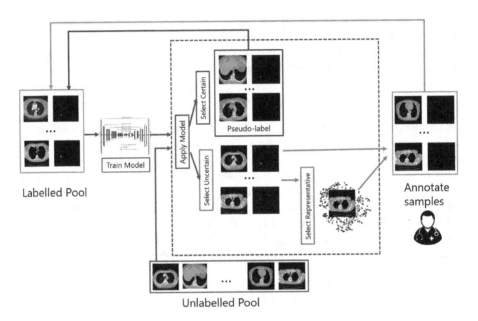

Fig. 2. Active learning setup showing our three active learning strategies in blue (uncertainty sampling), green (representativeness) and purple (pseudo-labelling). (Color figure online)

Baseline: Random Sampling: At every active learning iteration, four random patients are chosen from the unlabelled pool, and added to the labelled set.

AL Strategy 1: Uncertainty Sampling: At each iteration, the trained model is applied to the unlabelled slices to make T different predictions for each pixel, produced by T random dropout combinations in the bottleneck layer ($T = 3$, dropout $= 0.9$). In order to assign patient-level uncertainty scores, we compute the mean of the pixel-wise prediction variance across all pixels from all slices belonging to each patient. We add the four most uncertain patients to the labelled set. An example of a CT slice with associated uncertainty map is shown in Fig. 3.

AL Strategy 2: Representativeness: At each iteration, rather than simply selecting the most uncertain patients, we first designate the candidates as the U most uncertain patients ($U = 8$) using uncertainty scoring. For all unlabelled slices,

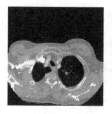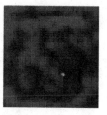

Fig. 3. Example scan slice with the corresponding labelling. From left to right: CT slice, GT annotation, Prediction, Uncertainty map. The prediction is from early training so the network has not yet learned to predict any part of the image with certainty, but the uncertainty for the nodule is over twice that of the background.

we then take the output of the U-Net bottleneck layer and apply principal component analysis with 10 components to produce a compressed representation. The R most representative candidates ($R = 4$) are selected by computing the mean cosine similarity between every slice in the candidate patient and every unlabelled slice. We add the R patients to the labelled set.

AL Strategy 3: Pseudo-Labelling: At each iteration, we select the C most *certain* patients ($C = 4$, measured by the lowest uncertainty scores) and add these patients to the labelled set with the soft probabilistic labels assigned by the network (pseudo-labels). Note that we require patients to have an uncertainty value below 0.001 to be considered for pseudo-labelling; this is to prevent low-quality labels being assigned when the model's predictions are uniformly poor for samples in the unlabelled pool (typically early on during training).

Each iteration consists of a training run as described in Sect. 3.2, starting from the pre-trained weights learned in the previous iteration. For all active learning experiments, initially the VGG U-Net was trained on all slices from 10 randomly chosen patients, and the remaining 252 patients were put into the unlabelled pool of data. For the purpose of the ablation study, we removed uncertainty scoring and employed representativeness alone (i.e., all unlabelled patients are candidates, not only the most uncertain), and pseudo-labelling alone (i.e., used in conjunction with random sampling rather than uncertainty sampling). To measure the upper bound i.e., the measure of achievable performance when all training data is used, the network was trained with all 262 patients.

4   Results

Figures 4 and 5 show the results. To capture the variation in the speed of the convergence, each strategy was run with 8 random seeds, each time randomly varying the initialisation conditions i.e., using different network weights and a different subset of 10 labelled patients from the training set (training, validation and test sets were kept fixed). The seeds were kept the same between approaches. In order to estimate the network performance at each active learning iteration, we compute the average precision-recall (PR) score using the test set. In the

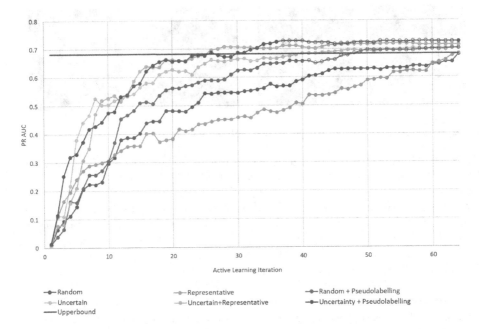

Fig. 4. Graph of the mean PR score (of 8 runs) for every strategy at each iteration. The full labelled training dataset is shown in red. (Color figure online)

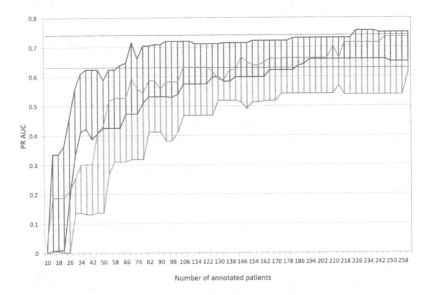

Fig. 5. Graph of the minimum and maximum PR score (of 8 runs) at each iteration for uncertainty sampling (blue) vs random sampling (grey). The full labelled training dataset is shown in red. (Color figure online)

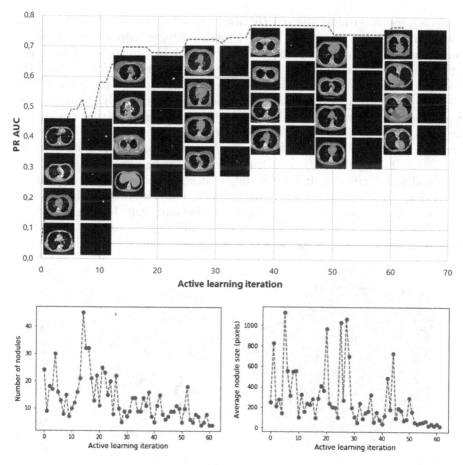

Fig. 6. Illustration of emergent selection policy for one training run of the uncertainty sampling strategy. Top: Graph showing a random slice from each of the 4 patients selected at each iteration. Bottom: Plots of the average number and size of nodules at each iteration (across the batch of 4 scans).

case of pseudo-labelling, for most runs, the unlabelled data was all added to the labelled pool as either true labels (through uncertainty selection, with or without representativeness) or pseudo-labels by around 40 iterations. In Fig. 4, for ease of visualisation, we extrapolate the final metric for each run up to the full 63 iterations. We note that dips are evident in the graphs, denoting worse performance from one iteration to the next, despite the fact that we retain the best weights on the validation set at each iteration. This occurs because the binary cross-entropy metric used to judge the best weights is not completely correlated with our evaluation metric of average precision-recall score (which is too computationally expensive for use within training). Below we analyse the results for each active learning method.

Uncertainty Sampling: Whilst there is large variation between the experiment runs (so performance is highly dependent on the initial random set of training patients), the uncertainty-based active learning methods almost always perform better than random sampling. In fact, these strategies appear on average to outperform the fully labelled dataset. To gain insight into the selection policy of the uncertainty sampling, in Fig. 6 we show a random slice from each of the four patients selected at each iteration for a single run. At the beginning of the training run, patients with large nodules were selected. By the end of the training run, patients with smaller nodules, frequently close to the lung border, were selected. We observe that this behaviour resembles a curriculum learning strategy, which makes an interesting emergent counterpoint to the hand-designed curriculum learning strategies such as has been previously demonstrated for lung nodule detection [9]. It is interesting that uncertainty sampling appears to outperform training with the fully labelled dataset, and we theorise that a better minimum may be reached due to sample selection mimicking balanced sampling i.e., eagerly selecting samples along different axes of variation such as nodule size, position, and opacity; however, further investigation is required.

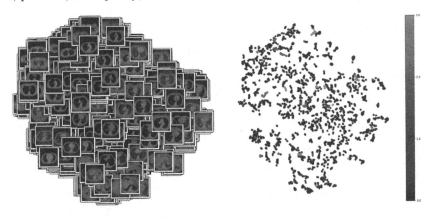

Fig. 7. 2D projection of slices within the representation space, using t-SNE [14]. The colours denote: 0 = Undiagnosed, 1 = Benign or non-malignant disease, 2 = Malignant primary lung cancer, 3 = Malignant metastatic cancer.

Representativeness: Sampling purely by representativeness is a poor strategy, however in combination with uncertainty sampling there is a small boost in performance. On visual inspection of the compressed bottleneck representation (see Fig. 7), we find that anatomical rather than pathological information is being captured. This is perhaps unsurprising given that the representation is derived from the U-Net bottleneck, which is bypassed by skip connections at many higher resolutions more suited to learning representations of small details such as lung nodules. It is possible that architectures such as proposed by Kohl *et al.* [11] would provide a more suitable representation. However, we also note that we deviated from the method of Yang *et al.* [22] in order to minimise computation time; we computed representativeness independently for each candidate patient, rather than for each set of candidate patients. This potentially means that the selected candidates will be correlated with one another, rather than representing variation across the whole unlabelled group; we reasoned that this effect would even out over the course of the active learning process as groups of candidates became certain one by one.

Pseudo-Labelling: Pseudo-labelling appears to be a promising strategy, although the additional benefit over uncertainty sampling is marginal. The approach here (following Gorriz *et al.* [7]) is a simple strategy that could be finessed by updating the pseudo-labels as the model improves during training, or returning samples to the unlabelled pool that become uncertain. Interesting alternative approaches have also recently emerged, such as the reinforcement learning method suggested by Park *et al.* [15] which claims substantial reductions in annotation effort for the task of lung nodule detection in chest X-Rays.

5   Conclusion

Using lung nodule segmentation as an exemplar focal pathology task, we have evaluated methods reported for other medical imaging tasks, showing that:

- Uncertainty sampling allows a model to be trained with less than half of the annotation effort but matching performance.
- Representativeness gives a small further improvement in combination with uncertainty sampling.
- Pseudolabelling gives small further improvements in combination with both random and uncertainty sampling strategies.

In future work, we plan to investigate better representations for small details such as the architecture recently proposed in [11] and more sophisticated pseudolabelling strategies such as [15]. However, we conclude that uncertainty sampling already offers significant annotation savings, with the practical feature that the pixelwise uncertainty maps could guide the annotator straight to the problematic regions in the scan. As large datasets become available which are suitable for diagnosis of focal pathologies, active learning techniques will be a valuable training tool.

References

1. Abraham, J.: Reduced lung cancer mortality with low-dose computed tomographic screening. Commun. Oncol. **8**(10), 441–442 (2011)
2. Armato III, S.G., et al.: Data from lidc-idri. the cancer imaging archive (2015)
3. Bank, D., Greenfeld, D., Hyams, G.: Improved training for self training by confidence assessments. In: Arai, K., Kapoor, S., Bhatia, R. (eds.) SAI 2018. AISC, vol. 858, pp. 163–173. Springer, Cham (2019). https://doi.org/10.1007/978-3-030-01174-1_13
4. Becker, N., et al.: Lung cancer mortality reduction by ldct screening-results from the randomised german lusi trial. International Journal of Cancer (2019)
5. Gal, Y., Ghahramani, Z.: Dropout as a bayesian approximation: representing model uncertainty in deep learning. In: international Conference on Machine Learning, pp. 1050–1059 (2016)

6. Golan, R., Jacob, C., Denzinger, J.: Lung nodule detection in ct images using deep convolutional neural networks. In: 2016 International Joint Conference on Neural Networks (IJCNN), pp. 243–250. IEEE (2016)
7. Gorriz, M., Carlier, A., Faure, E., Giro-i Nieto, X.: Cost-effective active learning for melanoma segmentation (2017). arXiv preprint arXiv:1711.09168
8. Hua, K.L., Hsu, C.H., Hidayati, S.C., Cheng, W.H., Chen, Y.J.: Computer-aided classification of lung nodules on computed tomography images via deep learning technique. Onco Targets Therapy **8**, 2015–2022 (2015)
9. Jesson, A., et al.: CASED: curriculum adaptive sampling for extreme data imbalance. In: Descoteaux, M., Maier-Hein, L., Franz, A., Jannin, P., Collins, D.L., Duchesne, S. (eds.) MICCAI 2017. LNCS, vol. 10435, pp. 639–646. Springer, Cham (2017). https://doi.org/10.1007/978-3-319-66179-7_73
10. Kingma, D.P., Ba, J.: Adam: a method for stochastic optimization (2014). arXiv preprint arXiv:1412.6980
11. Kohl, S.A., et al.: A hierarchical probabilistic u-net for modeling multi-scale ambiguities (2019). arXiv preprint arXiv:1905.13077
12. Lee, D.H.: Pseudo-label: the simple and efficient semi-supervised learning method for deep neural networks. In: Workshop on Challenges in Representation Learning, ICML. vol. 3, p. 2 (2013)
13. Lin, T.Y., Goyal, P., Girshick, R., He, K., Dollár, P.: Focal loss for dense object detection. IEEE Transactions on Pattern Analysis and Machine Intelligence (2018)
14. Maaten, L.V.D., Hinton, G.: Visualizing data using t-sne. J. Mach. Learn. Res. **9**, 2579–2605 (2008)
15. Park, S., Hwang, W., Jung, K.H.: Integrating reinforcement learning to self training for pulmonary nodule segmentation in chest x-rays. NeurIPS ML4 Health Workshop (2018)
16. Ronneberger, O., Fischer, P., Brox, T.: U-Net: convolutional networks for biomedical image segmentation. In: Navab, N., Hornegger, J., Wells, W.M., Frangi, A.F. (eds.) MICCAI 2015. LNCS, vol. 9351, pp. 234–241. Springer, Cham (2015). https://doi.org/10.1007/978-3-319-24574-4_28
17. Segal, R., Miller, K., Jemal, A.: Cancer statistics (2018). https://www.ncbi.nlm.nih.gov/pubmed/29313949
18. Settles, B.: Active learning literature survey. University of Wisconsin-Madison Department of Computer Sciences, Technical report (2009)
19. Simonyan, K., Zisserman, A.: Very deep convolutional networks for large-scale image recognition (2014). arXiv preprint arXiv:1409.1556
20. Smith, L.N.: Cyclical learning rates for training neural networks. In: 2017 IEEE Winter Conference on Applications of Computer Vision (WACV), pp. 464–472. IEEE (2017)
21. Wang, K., Zhang, D., Li, Y., Zhang, R., Lin, L.: Cost-effective active learning for deep image classification. IEEE Trans. Circ. Syst. Video Technol. **27**(12), 2591–2600 (2016)
22. Yang, L., Zhang, Y., Chen, J., Zhang, S., Chen, D.Z.: Suggestive annotation: a deep active learning framework for biomedical image segmentation. In: Descoteaux, M., Maier-Hein, L., Franz, A., Jannin, P., Collins, D.L., Duchesne, S. (eds.) MICCAI 2017. LNCS, vol. 10435, pp. 399–407. Springer, Cham (2017). https://doi.org/10.1007/978-3-319-66179-7_46

Robust Registration of Statistical Shape Models for Unsupervised Pathology Annotation

Dana Rahbani[✉], Andreas Morel-Forster, Dennis Madsen, Marcel Lüthi, and Thomas Vetter

Department of Mathematics and Computer Science,
University of Basel, Basel, Switzerland
`dana.rahbani@unibas.ch`

Abstract. We present a method to automatically label pathologies in volumetric medical data. Our solution makes use of a healthy statistical shape model to label pathologies in novel targets during model fitting. We achieve this using an EM algorithm: the E-step classifies surface points into pathological or healthy classes based on outliers in predicted correspondences, while the M-step performs probabilistic fitting of the statistical shape model to the healthy region. Our method is independent of pathology type or target anatomy, and can therefore be used for labeling different types of data. The method is able to detect pathologies with higher accuracy than standard robust detection algorithms, which we show using true positive rate and F1 scores. Furthermore, the method provides an estimate of the uncertainty of the synthesized label. The detection also directly improves surface reconstruction results, as shown by a decrease in the average and Hausdorff distances to ground truth. The method can be used for automated diagnosis or as a pre-processing step to accurately label large amounts of images.

Keywords: Statistical shape model · Label synthesis · Outlier detection · Robust non-rigid registration · EM algorithm

1 Introduction

Automatic labeling of biomedical data remains a necessity, whether for diagnosis in health-care or image annotation in datasets. This is especially the case for pathology labeling in volumetric data such as CT or MR images, where there are time, cost, and error constraints on getting expert labels. One main challenge for automatic labeling is the extreme variation which can be seen across pathologies. This limits the ability to generalize labeling algorithms across imaging domains or even within the same pathology type.

Algorithms that rely on generative methods assume there is an underlying model which can be used to analyze an image. One example is a statistical shape model (SSM), which is a linear parametric model of shape variation.

© Springer Nature Switzerland AG 2019
L. Zhou et al. (Eds.): LABELS 2019/HAL-MICCAI 2019/CuRIOUS 2019, LNCS 11851, pp. 13–21, 2019.
https://doi.org/10.1007/978-3-030-33642-4_2

SSMs can generalize well to represent novel instances within the same shape family. For example, an SSM built from healthy mandibles can be used to extract information about a novel mandible extracted from CT, such as location of teeth. However, the extreme variation problem also prevents the direct application of SSMs to pathological data, mainly because of unavailable correspondences needed for model building and fitting. Solutions usually involve disease-specific models [19] or handcrafted pathology features [12], but this is not always possible given limited data and intra-disease pathology variations.

We show how SSMs built from healthy anatomies can be exploited to perform pathology labeling in novel images. We treat pathology labeling as an outlier detection step in our proposed robust non-rigid registration algorithm. Outliers are all SSM points without a corresponding point in the target and vice versa. Our work extends combined fitting and segmentation with the EM-algorithm [2,5] to outlier detection on surfaces. We avoid pathology-specific modeling of features by introducing a probabilistic metric which does not depend on imaging modality or pathology type. The metric evaluates the target reconstruction and learns to perform unsupervised classification of individual data points into shape or pathology. The metric we implement is a probabilistic extension of a double-projection distance used in the iterative closest points (ICP) algorithm [1,16], explained in detail in Sect. 3.1. Our main contributions are:

1. an unsupervised-learning and probabilistic approach to label surfaces extracted from biomedical images as healthy or pathological
2. a robust registration algorithm for fitting SSMs to pathological data

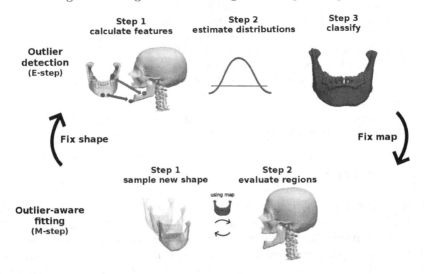

Fig. 1. Proposed pipeline for label synthesis and reconstruction. The input is an unlabeled pathological target surface. The outputs are the reconstruction, the label map and the estimated distributions. They are obtained by iterating between outlier detection (E-step) and outlier-aware fitting (M-step). The label map splits the reference topology into: healthy-region to be used in SSM fitting (blue) and outlier-region to be ignored by the SSM (red). (Color figure online)

2   Related Work

Given a dataset, the goal of outlier detection is to distinguish extreme values that are statistically relevant from those due to measurement errors [7]. A method can do so robustly if it has a high "breakdown point", a value which describes the number of outliers that can be present in a dataset before an algorithm fails [13]. For SSMs, outliers are model points which do not match their counterparts in a novel target. Approaches have been implemented to handle outliers:

Registration. In the trimmed ICP method (TrICP) [1], the robust Least Trimmed Squares algorithm is used in surface alignment. Other approaches for rigid registration of 3D surfaces with outliers make use of surface feature descriptors to match regions in correspondence [6]. However, we aim at non-rigid registration with missing or added data, which remains a difficult challenge. Non-rigid registration of point sets with outliers has been addressed in an extension to robust point matching [3] and in coherent point drift [15]. Instead of enforcing regularization on the allowed deformation fields as they do, we obtain deformation likelihoods directly from the SSM shape prior. In addition, outliers in our case include highly unlikely points under the shape prior instead of only missing or additional points in the set.

SSM-Based Approaches. Outlier detection for SSMs is a pre-processing step for building or fitting. Semantic patches are often introduced to narrow down the PCA space or reference topology [9,21]. SSMs have also been used for pathology segmentation from fitting errors [4]. Our method does not rely on a manual segmentation of the reference topology. We use fitting failures as in the second approach but go further by accounting for uncertainty in correspondences before pathology detection and improving reconstruction results.

Other Generative Approaches. Part-based models (PBMs) split SSMs into parts with a binary occurrence parameter [20], while Gaussian process morphable models (GPMMs) of shape and intensity [11,17] account for pathologies with local deformation kernels [10]. Recently, reconstruction errors from generative adversarial networks (GANs) have been used for pathology detection [18]. Our approach does not require local definitions of pathologies as PBMs or GPMMs do, nor does it depend on classification thresholds as GANs do.

3   Method

We extend the standard SSM fitting formulation with an additional segmentation of outliers. The segmentation takes the form of binary labels: one label for every point on the reference SSM topology. The labels separate two regions: an outlier-region and a healthy-region. SSM fitting is then restricted to the healthy-region. We formulate the detection and reconstruction steps together as a maximum a posteriori (MAP) estimation problem. The goal is to find the SSM shape and pose parameters θ and the point-level label map z that maximize the posterior distribution function given a target surface Γ:

$$P(\boldsymbol{\theta}, \boldsymbol{z} \mid \Gamma) \propto L(\Gamma \mid \boldsymbol{\theta}, \boldsymbol{z}) P(\boldsymbol{\theta}, \boldsymbol{z}) \qquad (1)$$

The likelihood evaluates the similarity of the SSM reconstruction $M(\boldsymbol{\theta})$ to the target Γ given a specific combination of $\boldsymbol{\theta}$ and $\boldsymbol{z}$, formulated as follows:

$$L(\Gamma \mid \boldsymbol{\theta}, \boldsymbol{z}) = \prod_{i \in n} l_h(M(\boldsymbol{\theta})_i, \Gamma_i)^{z_i} l_o(M(\boldsymbol{\theta})_i, \Gamma_i)^{1-z_i} \qquad (2)$$

The likelihood factors over the n reference topology points, since they are assumed to be independent. Every point i is evaluated by either the healthy-region distribution l_h or the outlier-region distribution l_o. The point label z_i indicates which of the two distributions should be used for the point i: if $z_i = 1$, then l_h is used, else $z_i = 0$ and l_o is used. The Euclidean distance is used to compare point i on the model surface $M(\boldsymbol{\theta})_i$ and its corresponding point on the target Γ_i.

Starting with a surface, the shape parameters $\boldsymbol{\theta}$, label map $\boldsymbol{z}$, and distributions l_h and l_o are unknown, making optimization intractable. We use an EM algorithm to solve this problem. In the E-step, we fix $\boldsymbol{\theta}$, learn the distributions l_h and l_o, then infer $\boldsymbol{z}$. In the M-step, we fix $\boldsymbol{z}$ and infer $\boldsymbol{\theta}$. The novel segmentation algorithm and the reconstruction strategy are presented in this section. Details on how to build SSMs can be found in Sect. 3 of [8] and Sect. 2 of [14].

3.1 Outlier Detection: Inferring the Label Map z

We want to infer the binary label map $\boldsymbol{z}$ defined on the domain of the SSM reference topology. Each of the n points has a label for one of two classes: healthy-region or outlier-region. In our examples, we consider the mandible with teeth as the healthy shape. Outliers could be holes from missing teeth, shape deformations from injuries or surgery, or artifacts.

Starting from Eq. 1, we fix the values of $\boldsymbol{\theta}$. We can then infer the labels which give the MAP solution. The unknown variables in the likelihood function are the distributions and the label map, both of which depend on the accuracy of the corresponding pairs. We propose a probabilistic interpretation of the distances between corresponding points to account for correspondence uncertainties, accomplished in the three steps below.

Determine Correspondences. A simple double-projection method proposed in an ICP-based alignment [16] is used. For every point of the SSM reference topology, we first find its closest point on the target, then project from this point back to the SSM. The output is a set of bidirectional correspondence pairs. Incorrect pairs are expected, not only because of this rough correspondence estimation approach, but also because in the beginning the fixed parameters $\boldsymbol{\theta}$ are far from the MAP solution.

Estimate Distributions. If the ground truth $\boldsymbol{\theta}$ and perfect correspondences were used, then we could expect l_h to be a univariate Gaussian with zero mean and standard deviation from reconstruction noise. However, since neither are available for pathological targets, l_h is a Gaussian distribution learned from the current double-projection distances. We assume a uniform distribution for l_o since the method is independent of pathology type. The likelihood is fixed at the value three standard deviations away from the mean of a healthy distribution, which we learn by fitting to 100 healthy shapes sampled from the SSM.

Infer Label Map. A point is considered an outlier if its double-projection distance has a higher likelihood of belonging to the outlier-region distribution than to the healthy-region distribution. We infer every z_i by choosing the label corresponding to the larger likelihood value. This is equivalent to maximizing the likelihood function in Eq. 2 with respect to z.

3.2   Outlier-Aware SSM Fitting: Inferring the SSM Parameters θ

To fit the SSM to the target, we need to maximize Eq. 1 with respect to the SSM parameters θ. To do so, we first fix the values of z obtained from the E-step. This leaves θ as the only remaining unknown in the likelihood Eq. 2. The prior on the shape parameters $P(\theta)$ is provided by the SSM. With this information, we can find θ by maximizing Eq. 1 using the approach in [14], which approximates the posterior distribution then takes the MAP solution as the best reconstruction.

4   Evaluation

We evaluate our method on a mandible SSM built from eight surfaces extracted from healthy CT scans. The meshes are registered with Gaussian process morphable models [11]. The healthy mandible SSM is built from the registered meshes using PCA. We generate pathological targets with known ground truth label maps and SSM parameters. For this, we sample shapes from the healthy model and deform or clip away parts of their surfaces. This ensures that the model is able to represent the target shape without pathologies and allows us to evaluate the effect of the labeling algorithm, instead of the SSM generalization ability, on the registration. This results in 25 test cases, two of which are shown in Fig. 2. We then apply the method on real data, with target surfaces extracted from CT images. Visualization is performed using *Scalismo*[1].

Added data   **Missing data**

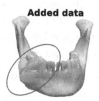 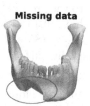

Fig. 2. Mandible shape with example pathologies circled in red. (Color figure online)

---

[1] https://scalismo.org.

Model fitting is performed for shape and pose parameters after rigid landmark alignment. Three approaches are compared: (1) standard SSM, which only performs reconstruction without segmentation, (2) robust SSM, which diminishes the effect of outliers based on the Huber Loss function with a 5 mm threshold, and (3) outlier-aware SSM. The threshold for the robust SSM is manually assigned because the learned threshold proved to be too large. For every outlier detection step, 1,000 iterations are taken in the fitting step. The entire process is repeated ten times as this empirically showed convergence by a constant healthy-region distribution. For comparison, 10,000 iterations are performed for the standard and robust SSMs.

Labeling Evaluation. Label maps are evaluated by the true positive rate (TPR) and the F1 scores compared to the ground truth labels. The TPR is the ratio of the number of true detected outlier points to the number of ground truth outlier points. It is used to give an idea of how much of the outlier region is detected. The F1 score is the harmonic mean of TPR and precision, where precision is the ratio of true detected outlier points to all detected outlier points. The F1 score is used to evaluate binary classification tasks with class imbalance. Figure 3 shows examples of the label maps for a missing data case. TPR and F1 scores in Table 1 reveal that the outlier-aware SSM outperforms the robust SSM.

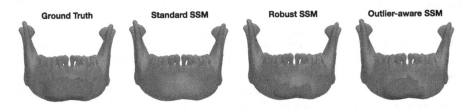

Fig. 3. Visual comparison of label maps projected onto the reference SSM topology: healthy-region (blue) and outlier-region (red). Pathology detection is not a feature of the standard SSM, which is why the entire topology is labeled as healthy. (Color figure online)

Reconstruction Evaluation. Reconstructions are evaluated by their Hausdorff and average distances to the ground truth healthy surface, seen in Table 1. There is a strong decrease in both distances when the outlier-aware SSM is used instead of the standard and robust SSMs. This is accredited to a closer reconstruction of the ground truth healthy surface in both the healthy and outlier regions.

Breakdown Point Evaluation. The breakdown point is defined as the fraction of points that can be outliers before the algorithm fails. We generate pathologies that cover an increasing fraction of the reference surface. The fitting degrades strongly if more than a third of the observed surface is pathological. Just before the breakdown point, we still reach an F1 score of 0.74 and an average distance of 1.08 mm.

Table 1. Labeling and fitting evaluations: mean values followed by standard deviations in parentheses. The mean values of the true positive rates (TPR) and F1 scores are best at 1, while those of the Hausdorff and Average distances (HD and AD) at 0 mm.

	Standard SSM (no labeling)	Robust SSM (thresholded labeling)	Outlier-aware SSM (probabilistic labeling)
TPR	–	0.39 (0.22)	**0.56 (0.22)**
F1	–	0.51 (0.27)	**0.68 (0.22)**
HD	4.48 (5.46)	6.07 (5.37)	**1.98 (0.89)**
AD	1.14 (0.51)	1.52 (0.49)	**0.88 (0.23)**

Label Uncertainty. We apply the algorithm to radius and mandible surfaces extracted from pathological CT images. Pathologies are regions of overgrowth for the radius and regions of missing teeth for the mandible, as seen in the targets in Fig. 4. We use a radius SSM built from 37 surfaces and mandible SSM from 8 surfaces as the models, all built from healthy CT images.

We use our proposed outlier-aware SSM to register and label the target surfaces and their reconstructions. Unlike the synthetic data case, surfaces extracted from real CT images by simple thresholding are not as clean. This can be seen for the mandible example in Fig. 4, where the cranium and the spine are parts of the input target surface. The proposed method can be applied on the surface with irrelevant data, without requiring user input other than the initial rigid alignment. We accomplish this by including both the model and target surfaces into the likelihood function, in Eq. 2. Using the distributions learned from step 2 of the E-step (Fig. 1) and the distances between the target and reconstruction, we can compute the uncertainty for the synthesized labels. The target and fitting

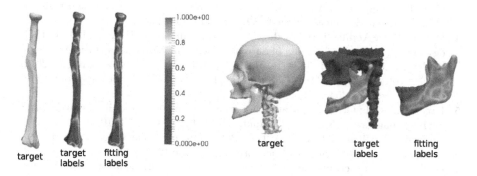

Fig. 4. Uncertainty in generated labels for target radius and skull surfaces, both extracted from pathological CT images. Pathology labels with high certainty are in red. Note that for the mandible example, we crop the target for computational purposes with a box from six landmarks. Given the remaining surface, the method is able to correctly locate irrelevant regions, as indicated by red labels on the cranium and spine. (Color figure online)

labels in Fig. 4 show the certainty levels for the generated pathology labels. Red indicates high certainty for the pathological label and blue for the healthy label.

5 Conclusion

Supervised pathology detection algorithms depend on expert labels or pathology thresholds. However, our proposed outlier-aware SSM is able to perform the detection given only a target surface without any further assumptions or user annotations. Pathology detection with our approach accomplishes higher true positive rates and F1 scores than classical robust statistics methods do. This results in a closer approximation of the ground truth healthy target, seen with reduction in the average distances, and also an uncertainty estimate on the synthesized labels. Our pipeline is non-specific to pathology type or imaging domain. This implies it can be used to point out regions of interest to clinicians or as a pre-processing step for training end-to-end classifiers. Future work will investigate other probabilistic metrics that can work alongside the distance-based one, as well as further testing of the method on current biomedical image segmentation challenges.

References

1. Chetverikov, D., Stepanov, D., Krsek, P.: Robust euclidean alignment of 3D point sets: the trimmed iterative closest point algorithm. Image Vis. Comput. **23**(3), 299–309 (2005)
2. Chitphakdithai, N., Duncan, J.S.: Non-rigid registration with missing correspondences in preoperative and postresection brain images. In: Jiang, T., Navab, N., Pluim, J.P.W., Viergever, M.A. (eds.) MICCAI 2010. LNCS, vol. 6361, pp. 367–374. Springer, Heidelberg (2010). https://doi.org/10.1007/978-3-642-15705-9_45
3. Chui, H., Rangarajan, A.: A new point matching algorithm for non-rigid registration. Comput. Vis. Image Underst. **89**(2–3), 114–141 (2003)
4. Dufour, P.A., Abdillahi, H., Ceklic, L., Wolf-Schnurrbusch, U., Kowal, J.: Pathology hinting as the combination of automatic segmentation with a statistical shape model. In: Ayache, N., Delingette, H., Golland, P., Mori, K. (eds.) MICCAI 2012. LNCS, vol. 7512, pp. 599–606. Springer, Heidelberg (2012). https://doi.org/10.1007/978-3-642-33454-2_74
5. Egger, B., et al.: Occlusion-aware 3D morphable models and an illumination prior for face image analysis. Int. J. Comput. Vis. **126**, 1269–1287 (2018)
6. Gelfand, N., Mitra, N.J., Guibas, L.J., Pottmann, H.: Robust global registration. In: Symposium on Geometry Processing, vol. 2, p. 5 (2005)
7. Grubbs, F.E.: Procedures for detecting outlying observations in samples. Technometrics **11**(1), 1–21 (1969)
8. Heimann, T., Meinzer, H.P.: Statistical shape models for 3D medical image segmentation: a review. Med. Image Anal. **13**(4), 543–563 (2009)
9. Lüthi, M., Albrecht, T., Vetter, T.: Building shape models from lousy data. In: Yang, G.-Z., Hawkes, D., Rueckert, D., Noble, A., Taylor, C. (eds.) MICCAI 2009. LNCS, vol. 5762, pp. 1–8. Springer, Heidelberg (2009). https://doi.org/10.1007/978-3-642-04271-3_1

10. Lüthi, M., Forster, A., Gerig, T., Vetter, T.: Shape modeling using Gaussian process morphable models. In: Statistical Shape and Deformation Analysis, pp. 165–191. Elsevier (2017)
11. Lüthi, M., Gerig, T., Jud, C., Vetter, T.: Gaussian process morphable models. IEEE Trans. Pattern Anal. Mach. Intell. **40**(8), 1860–1873 (2018)
12. Madabhushi, A., Lee, G.: Image analysis and machine learning in digital pathology: challenges and opportunities (2016)
13. Meer, P., Mintz, D., Rosenfeld, A., Kim, D.Y.: Robust regression methods for computer vision: a review. Int. J. Comput. Vis. **6**(1), 59–70 (1991)
14. Morel-Forster, A., Gerig, T., Lüthi, M., Vetter, T.: Probabilistic fitting of active shape models. In: Reuter, M., Wachinger, C., Lombaert, H., Paniagua, B., Lüthi, M., Egger, B. (eds.) ShapeMI 2018. LNCS, vol. 11167, pp. 137–146. Springer, Cham (2018). https://doi.org/10.1007/978-3-030-04747-4_13
15. Myronenko, A., Song, X.: Point set registration: coherent point drift. IEEE Trans. Pattern Anal. Mach. Intell. **32**(12), 2262–2275 (2010)
16. Pajdla, T., Van Gool, L.: Matching of 3-D curves using semi-differential invariants. In: Proceedings of IEEE International Conference on Computer Vision, pp. 390–395. IEEE (1995)
17. Reyneke, C., Thusini, X., Douglas, T., Vetter, T., Mutsvangwa, T.: Construction and validation of image-based statistical shape and intensity models of bone. In: 2018 3rd Biennial South African Biomedical Engineering Conference (SAIBMEC), pp. 1–4. IEEE (2018)
18. Schlegl, T., Seeböck, P., Waldstein, S.M., Schmidt-Erfurth, U., Langs, G.: Unsupervised anomaly detection with generative adversarial networks to guide marker discovery. In: Niethammer, M., Styner, M., Aylward, S., Zhu, H., Oguz, I., Yap, P.-T., Shen, D. (eds.) IPMI 2017. LNCS, vol. 10265, pp. 146–157. Springer, Cham (2017). https://doi.org/10.1007/978-3-319-59050-9_12
19. Thompson, P.M., Woods, R.P., Mega, M.S., Toga, A.W.: Mathematical/computational challenges in creating deformable and probabilistic atlases of the human brain. Hum. Brain Mapp. **9**(2), 81–92 (2000)
20. Toews, M., Arbel, T.: A statistical parts-based model of anatomical variability. IEEE Trans. Med. Imaging **26**(4), 497–508 (2007)
21. Yokota, F., Okada, T., Takao, M., Sugano, N., Tada, Y., Tomiyama, N., Sato, Y.: Automated CT segmentation of diseased hip using hierarchical and conditional statistical shape models. In: Mori, K., Sakuma, I., Sato, Y., Barillot, C., Navab, N. (eds.) MICCAI 2013. LNCS, vol. 8150, pp. 190–197. Springer, Heidelberg (2013). https://doi.org/10.1007/978-3-642-40763-5_24

XiangyaDerm: A Clinical Image Dataset of Asian Race for Skin Disease Aided Diagnosis

Bin Xie[1,2], Xiaoyu He[1], Shuang Zhao[2,3], Yi Li[1,2], Juan Su[3],
Xinyu Zhao[1], Yehong Kuang[3], Yong Wang[1,2], and Xiang Chen[3(✉)]

[1] School of Automation, Central South University, Changsha, China
hexiaoyu@csu.edu.cn
[2] Mobile Health Ministry of Education - China Mobile Joint Laboratory,
Central South University, Changsha, China
{xiebin, shuangxy}@csu.edu.cn
[3] Department of Dermatology, Xiangya Hospital, Central South University,
Changsha, China
chenxiangck@126.com

Abstract. Skin disease is a quite common disease of human beings, which has been found in all races and ages. It seriously affects people's quality of life or even endangers people's lives. In this paper, we propose a large-scale, Asian-dominated dataset of skin diseases with bounding box labels, namely Xiangya-Derm. It contains 107,565 clinical images, covering 541 types of skin diseases. Each image in this dataset is labeled by professional doctors. As far as we know, this dataset is the largest clinical image dataset of Asian skin diseases used in Computer Aided Diagnosis (CAD) system worldwide. We compare the classification results of several advanced Convolutional Neural Networks (CNNs) on this dataset. InceptionResNetV2 is the best one for 80 skin disease classification whose Top-1 and Top-3 accuracies can reach 0.588 and 0.764, which proves the usefulness of the proposed benchmark dataset, and gives the baseline performance on it. The cross-test experiment with Derm101 shows us that the CNN model has a very different test effect on different ethnic datasets. Therefore, to build a skin disease CAD system with high performance and stability, we recommend to establish a specific dataset of skin diseases for different regions and races.

Keywords: Skin disease · Clinical image dataset · Computer Aided Diagnosis

1 Introduction

Skin disease is a very common disease of human beings, which has been found in all races and ages [1]. Skin diseases can bring many troubles to patients, such as itching, bleeding and so on, which seriously affect people's quality of life or even endanger lives. Early diagnosis of skin diseases is very important, which can make patients get correct treatment as soon as possible and arrest the growth of the disease. However, due to the

---

Electronic supplementary material The online version of this chapter (https://doi.org/10.1007/978-3-030-33642-4_3) contains supplementary material, which is available to authorized users.

L. Zhou et al. (Eds.): LABELS 2019/HAL-MICCAI 2019/CuRIOUS 2019, LNCS 11851, pp. 22–31, 2019.
https://doi.org/10.1007/978-3-030-33642-4_3

limited medical knowledge of patients and the disparity of medical resources, such case of delaying the timing of diagnosis occurs from time to time. The emergence of the CAD system can help us solve these problems to a certain extent. Early studies on skin diseases CAD system are mostly focused on dermoscopic images [2, 3]. This is because they focus more on lesions than clinical images with uniform illumination and less noise. In fact, dermoscopic-based diagnosis of skin diseases has some limitations in promotion, such as high fees and less convenience. In recent years, some researchers begin to pay more attention to clinical images [4–7]. Their works' datasets were mainly collected in Europe and America. The lack of a specific Asian skin disease dataset has become a major hindrance to the study of skin disease diagnostic system.

Convolution neural network is very popular in the field of feature learning and object recognition in recent years. Many studies from ImageNet's large-scale visual challenge [8–11] (ILSVRC) [12] show that the most advanced CNN has exceeded human level in object classification tasks. However, the classification performance of CNN sometimes depends too much on the dataset. We designed cross-test experiments to study this problem.

The contributions of this paper are summarized below. Firstly, a large-scale, Asian-dominated dataset of skin diseases is proposed. Secondly, in order to evaluate the usefulness of our dataset, we give the baseline performance on this dataset. Finally, through cross-test experiments between different datasets, we draw the conclusion that the skin disease diagnosis systems should be setup on specific datasets. We have good reason to believe that the dataset proposed in this paper is very urgent and meaningful for the research of skin disease diagnosis.

2 Related Work

Esteva et al. [13] achieved good recognition rate between keratinocytic carcinoma and benign seborrheic keratosis, malignant melanoma and benign nevus using Inception V3 CNN architecture on Dermofit and ISIC datasets., reaching the level of human dermatologists. This landmark research has attracted wide attention, especially in the field of AI in skin diseases.

Sun et al. [4] introduced datasets SD-198 and SD-128 based on DermQuest (now DermQuest is merged into Derm101). Several kinds of manual features extraction methods and deep learning methods are compared on these two datasets. SD-198 contains 198 different diseases, a total of 6,584 images. SD-128 is a subset of SD-198, ensuring that each class has more than 20 images. This benchmark dataset encourages many studies about visual skin disease classification. However, they classify 198 or 128 categories of skin diseases using a dataset of 6,584 images, which seems too small for CNN because the average number of training sets and test sets for per category is only 50.

Liao et al. [7] collected their dataset from 6 public dermatology atlas websites: AtlasDerm, Danderm, Derma, DermIS, Dermnet and DermQuest. They use CNNs for disease-targeted and lesion-targeted classifications and draw a conclusion that the classification method with lesion tags can get better performance. Their work is very meaningful both in methods and datasets. Next, we will briefly introduce the datasets mentioned above.

Dermofit dataset is provided by researchers at the University of Edinburgh in the United Kingdom. This dataset is of high quality and widely used by researchers, but it is not free available. Dermofit includes 10 types of skin diseases: actinic keratosis, basal cell carcinoma, melanocytic nevus, seborrheic keratosis, squamous cell carcinoma, intraepithelial carcinoma, pyogenic granuloma, hemangioma, dermatofibroma and malignant melanoma., but the total number of images is only about 1,300.

ISIC dataset comes from the International Skin Imaging Collaboration (ISIC), which aims to promote the diagnostic ability of skin image data. The dataset contains 23,906 images of 16 types of skin diseases, including both dermoscopic images and clinical images, with high quality and no watermarks. Each image in this dataset contains the tags of patient's age, gender, and lesion size. However, there are only 100 clinical images in the dataset, including 37 melanomas, 40 basal cell carcinomas and 23 squamous cell carcinomas, which is too small for the training of deep learning methods.

Derm101 is a website for providing clinicians with high-caliber and up-to-date content. It also provides a clinical dataset of 22,979 images of 525 types of skin diseases, containing labels both for disease diagnosis and lesion location, without watermarks on the image too. Fortunately, we have obtained permission from the Derm101 team to use their images for research purposes. Later, we organized experiments related to this dataset.

Dermnet is called to be the largest independent photo dermatology source dedicated to online medical education. The image library of Dermnet is nearly 18,974 images, 626 types of skin diseases. However, each image in this dataset has only the label of the disease diagnosis, without any other labels.

DermIS is a free dataset website built by the University of Heidelberg, Germany. There are 7,172 images in this database, which are divided into 735 categories. Each image in this dataset has regular disease diagnosis labels as well as the text descriptions of lesion location, race and age. The drawback of this dataset is that the number of images in each class is not large and the image is watermarked.

AtlasDerm is a Brazilian dataset website. There are 9,503 images and 534 categories of skin diseases. Most of the data are mainly about Brazilians in South America. Each image in this dataset has only the label of disease diagnosis, and the image is watermarked.

Danderm is a clinical image data collection website of skin diseases from Denmark. There are 1,110 images and 91 types of skin diseases. Most of the patients collected in this dataset are white races, only have the label of disease diagnosis, and contain the watermarking occlusion.

In a conclusion, we summarize the above datasets into Table 1. It can be seen from Table 1 that there are some obvious defects in the existing skin disease datasets:

(1) The current datasets are mainly based on Caucasian and Black races in Europe and America, and the large-scale standardized dataset of Asian has not been reported before. Obviously, there are differences in the incidence of skin diseases, disease characteristics, and the background of skin color among different races.
(2) Most of the images currently available in the dataset are watermarked, which may cause interference in the identification and analysis of skin lesions.

Table 1. Comparisons of clinical skin disease datasets.

Dataset	Classes	Amount	Region	Watermarking?	Available?
Dermofit	10	1,300	The UK	No	No
ISIC	16	23,906	Europe	No	Yes
Derm101	525	22,979	The US	No	Yes
Dermnet	626	18,974	Europe	Yes	Yes
DermIS	735	7,172	Germany	Yes	Yes
AtlasDerm	534	9,503	Brazil	Yes	Yes
Danderm	91	1,110	Denmark	Yes	Yes
Ours	541	107,565	China	No	Yes

In this paper, we establish a large-scale, Asian-dominated clinical image dataset of skin diseases, and carries out researches on it. The statistical data of XiangyaDerm is also presented in Table 1 for comparison with other public datasets. Our dataset will be publicly released for research purposes to the internet soon after, and the future update information could be found in this URL, http://airl.csu.edu.cn/xiangyaderm.

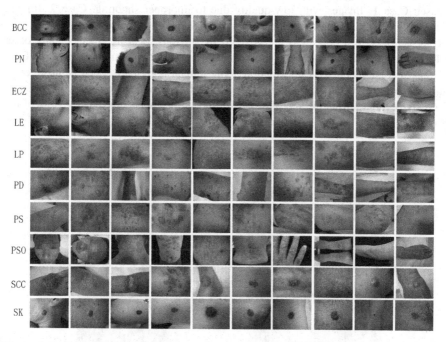

Fig. 1. Some sample images in XiangyaDerm. Each line from top to bottom are clinical images of basal cell carcinoma (BCC), pigmented nevus (PN), eczema (ECZ), lupus erythematosus (LE), lichen planus (LP), pemphigoid (PD), pemphigus (PS), psoriasis (PSO), squamous cell carcinoma (SCC), and seborrheic keratosis (SK).

3   Dataset

3.1   Data Acquisition and Cleaning

The collection of XiangyaDerm was approved by the Ethics Committee of Xiangya Hospital of Central South University, and informed consent was obtained from all participants. All clinical images were taken by dermatologists from Xiangya Hospital under standard illumination using four different cameras: SONY DSC-HX50 (350dpi), CANON IXUS 50 (180dpi), NIKON D40 (300dpi), NIKON COOLPIX L340 (300dpi), corresponding resolution of 3,888 × 5,184, 1,944 × 2,592, 2,000 × 3,008, 3,864 × 5,152. Finally, a total dataset of 47,075 images was obtained, covering 541 skin diseases, accounted for almost 99% of the incidence of skin diseases. The diagnostic labels for each image are validated by the gold standard of pathology and are supported by the patient's full medical history. We show some sample images in Fig. 1. We can see that these images are with high image quality, simple background, and focus mainly on the typical skin lesions. For example, we chose the images of pemphigus with bullae instead of papules and plaques.

The data cleaning process is also accomplished by dermatologists from Xiangya Hospital. Five categories of images are removed in this process to obtain a clean dataset: Case 1: Images with low-quality due to improper shooting. Case 2: Images incorrectly labeled which confirmed to be inconsistent with the patient's medical history. Case 3: Skin lesion areas are covered by obvious local treatment or any other colored residues, which may have serious adverse effects on the training process. Case 4: Images contains obvious information about human body parts, such as nose, eyes, hair and so on, which can also interfere with the subsequent recognition. Case 5: Excessive exudate, which leads to the loss of the surface appearance and texture of the disease.

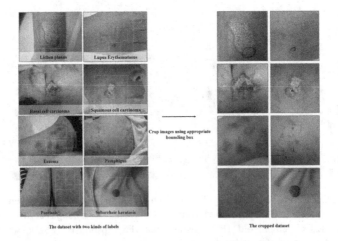

Fig. 2. The data annotation and cropping process for XiangyaDerm.

3.2 Data Annotation and Cropping

The annotation process is completed by 20 professional dermatologists, with more than 5 years of clinical work experience. These doctors were divided into two separate groups, each labeled half of the images and then cross-checked the other half. The task of annotation is to use labeling, an open source image annotation software, to mark the typical lesion areas on the picture, that is, to represent the lesion area with a bounding box.

The cropping process uses the coordinates of the bounding box on the image to save that part of the image. As shown in Fig. 2, after the cropping operation, not only the complex background of the skin image is removed, but also the amount of dataset is increased, since a picture may have several typical isolated skin lesions.

Eventually, the data volume of our dataset increased from 44,108 to 107,565, covering 541 categories of skin diseases, and the images were more concentrated on skin lesions. The largest amount of data in our dataset is psoriasis, 67,066 images, accounting for 62% of the total dataset. This is mainly because the dermatology department of Xiangya Hospital is a special outpatient department of psoriasis, and there are many patients with psoriasis every year. In addition to psoriasis, the data distribution of the remaining 540 skin diseases is shown in Fig. 3, with the horizontal and vertical axes representing the disease and its corresponding data volume.

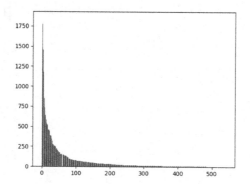

Fig. 3. The distribution of the final proposed dataset except psoriasis.

4 Experiment

4.1 80-Classification Experiment on XiangyaDerm

In order to evaluate the performances of different CNNs on this dataset and prove the usefulness of it, we select 4 mainstream CNN architectures, including InceptionV3 [14], InceptionResNetV2 [15], DenseNet121 [16] and Xception [17] to classify 80 common skin diseases. We select 80 kinds of skin diseases in our dataset whose amount of data is more than 100, and remove the parts whose amount of data is more than 1,000 in order to balance the chose 80 skin disease. The specific number of these 80 diseases in this experiment can be seen in the submitted supplementary files, which name is "appendix.pdf".

In this experiment, our dataset is randomly divided into training set and test set in a ratio of 3:1. The whole training process was completed on 3 graphic cards of NVIDIA TITAN Xp. The image input size for InceptionV3, InceptionResNetV2 and Xception are both $299 \times 299 \times 3$ and for Densenet121 is $224 \times 224 \times 3$. We kept the rest of the experimental conditions consistent, for example, setting the same pre-trained weights on ImageNet dataset, max training epochs 5000, basic learning rates 0.001, batch size 25, optimizer Adam, and the loss function categorical cross entropy. By organizing 4-fold cross validation experiments, we summarize the average values of the experimental results as shown in Table 2 and Fig. 4.

Table 2. Recognition rate of 80-classification experiment.

Method	InceptionV3	DenseNet121	Xception	InceptionResNetV2
Top1 ACC	0.470	0.494	0.523	0.588
Top3 ACC	0.671	0.696	0.707	0.764

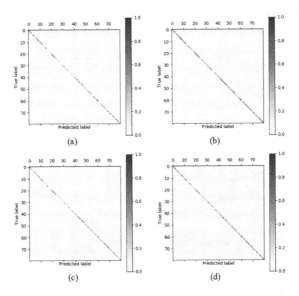

Fig. 4. Confusion matrices of 80-classification experiments: (a), (b), (c) and (d) represent test results for InceptionV3, DenseNet121, Xception, and InceptionResNetV2, respectively.

From the confusion matrix shown in Fig. 4, we can see these 4 CNNs all have good performances. We can see that the dark green area of the confusion matrix is mainly distributed on the diagonal line, while the color of other areas is relatively light. It shows that most of the 80 skin diseases can be effectively distinguished by the adopted CNNs, except for a few indistinguishable diseases. However, it does not mean that there are problems with our dataset or CNNs, which just shows that the diagnosis of these skin diseases based only on clinical images still faces challenges.

As we can see from Table 2, we can draw a preliminary conclusion that InceptionResNetV2 could get better performance over other 3 networks in the 80-classification experiment on XiangyaDerm. Note that our goal is not to find the best network for recognition, but to verify the usefulness of our proposed datasets and give a baseline performance on it.

4.2   6-Classification Cross-Test of Derm101 and XiangyaDerm

As mentioned earlier in this paper, we have been successfully approved by the Derm101 team to use their images for research purposes. The objective of this experiment is to obtain the cross-test performance of datasets between different races. We chose 6 common diseases witch high incidence and both occurred in Derm101 and XiangyaDerm whose amount is more than 100, including Basal Cell Carcinoma, Epidermoid Cyst, Psoriasis, Rosacea, Seborrheic Keratosis and Stasis Dermatitis. To balance each category in the datasets we took 100 images from each category and formed two sub-databases, namely Derm101-6 and Xiangya-6. Another dataset is Mix-6, which is a dataset composed of Derm101-6 and Xiangya-6.

As for the experimental settings, we used InceptionResNetV2, which is the best performing CNN in 80-classification experiment, to do cross-test on Derm101-6, Xiangya-6, and Mix-6. The loss function, batch size and other parameter settings are kept the same as the previous experiment. The cross-test here means that the model trained on one dataset is tested on the other two datasets. The test results obtained in this experiment are shown in Table 3 and Fig. 5.

Table 3. Recognition rate of 6-classification experiment.

	Test on Derm101-6	Test on Xiangya-6
Train on Derm101-6	0.800	0.193
Train on Xiangya-6	0.213	0.720
Train on Mix-6	0.671	0.621

As we can see from (a) and (d) of Fig. 5, the dark squares are concentrated on the diagonal lines which shows that the classification of each disease is also good, while the accuracy is much worse when we exchange the test sets. From Table 3, from the comparison between (a) (d) and (b) (c), we can see that the model trained and test on the same dataset has a better performance than the cross-test ones. As we can see from (a) and (d) of Fig. 5. Comparing (e) (a) (c) and (f) (b) (d), we can easily find that the model trained on the mixed training dataset reached a better performance than training and test on a totally different dataset but worse than training and test on a same dataset.

From this, we can see that the cross-test performance of classification models between different races is not good. Through communication with professional dermatologists, we understand that there are differences in the incidence of skin diseases, disease manifestations, and skin color among different races, which can lead to the failure of classification models. Therefore, to build a skin disease CAD system with high performance and stability, we recommend to establish a specific dataset of skin diseases for different regions and races.

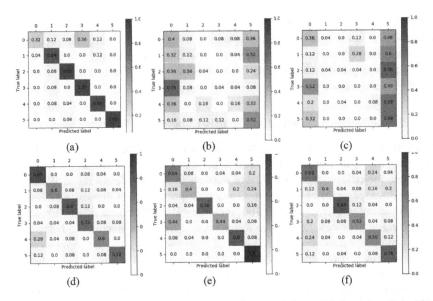

Fig. 5. Confusion matrices of 6-classification experiment: (a) Derm101-6 training Derm101-6 test, (b) Derm101-6 training Xiangya-6 test, (c) Xiangya-6 training Derm101-6 test, (d) Xiangya-6 training Xiangya-6 test, (e) Mix-6 training Derm101-6 test, (f) Mix-6 training Xiangya-6 test.

5 Conclusion

In this paper, we propose a clinical image dataset for Asian race's skin disease diagnosis system. It contains 107,565 images, ranging from 541 categories. Each image is confirmed by a disease label and is marked by a specialist with bounding boxes. Our experiments demonstrate the classification performances of the current state-of-the-art CNN architectures and demonstrate its usability as a benchmark dataset for the diagnosis of skin diseases. Moreover, we have also proved that it is necessary to construct a specific dataset of skin diseases for different regions and races through the cross-test experiments. The XiangyaDerm proposed in this paper can effectively promote the research and application of Asian skin disease diagnosis, and is also a useful supplement to global skin data.

References

1. Hay, R.J., Johns, N.E., Williams, H.C., et al.: The global burden of skin disease in 2010: an analysis of the prevalence and impact of skin conditions. J. Invest. Dermatol. **134**(6), 1527–1534 (2014)
2. Gonzalez-Castro, V., Debayle, J., Wazaefi, Y., et al.: Automatic classification of skin lesions using color mathematical morphology-based texture descriptors. In: Twelfth International Conference on Quality Control by Artificial Vision 2015. International Society for Optics and Photonics, vol. 9534, p. 953409 (2015)

3. Badano, A., Revie, C., Casertano, A., et al.: Consistency and standardization of color in medical imaging: a consensus report. J. Digit. Imaging **28**(1), 41–52 (2015)
4. Sun, X., Yang, J., Sun, M., Wang, K.: A benchmark for automatic visual classification of clinical skin disease images. In: Leibe, B., Matas, J., Sebe, N., Welling, M. (eds.) ECCV 2016. LNCS, vol. 9910, pp. 206–222. Springer, Cham (2016). https://doi.org/10.1007/978-3-319-46466-4_13
5. Yang, J., Sun, X., Jie, L., et al.: Clinical skin lesion diagnosis using representations inspired by dermatologist criteria. In: IEEE Conference on Computer Vision and Pattern Recognition, p. 11 (2018)
6. Liao, H.: A deep learning approach to universal skin disease classification. University of Rochester Department of Computer Science, CSC (2016)
7. Liao, H., Li, Y., Luo, J.: Skin disease classification versus skin lesion characterization: achieving robust diagnosis using multi-label deep neural networks. In: 2016 23rd International Conference on Pattern Recognition (ICPR), pp. 355–360. IEEE (2016)
8. Deng, J., Dong, W., Socher, R., et al.: Imagenet: a large-scale hierarchical image database. In: IEEE Conference on Computer Vision and Pattern Recognition, 2009. CVPR 2009, pp. 248–255. IEEE (2009)
9. Sermanet, P., Eigen, D., Zhang, X., et al.: Overfeat: integrated recognition, localization and detection using convolutional networks. arXiv preprint arXiv:1312.6229 (2013)
10. Ioffe, S., Szegedy, C.: Batch normalization: accelerating deep network training by reducing internal covariate shift. arXiv preprint arXiv:1502.03167 (2015)
11. Szegedy, C., Liu, W., Jia, Y., et al.: Going deeper with convolutions. In: Proceedings of the IEEE Conference on Computer Vision and Pattern Recognition, pp. 1–9 (2015)
12. Russakovsky, O., Deng, J., Su, H., et al.: Imagenet large scale visual recognition challenge. Int. J. Comput. Vis. **115**(3), 211–252 (2015)
13. Esteva, A., Kuprel, B., Novoa, R.A., et al.: Dermatologist-level classification of skin cancer with deep neural networks. Nature **542**(7639), 115 (2017)
14. Szegedy, C., Vanhoucke, V., Ioffe, S., et al.: Rethinking the inception architecture for computer vision. In: Proceedings of the IEEE Conference on Computer Vision and Pattern Recognition, pp. 2818–2826 (2016)
15. Szegedy, C., Ioffe, S., Vanhoucke, V., et al.: Inception-v4, inception-resnet and the impact of residual connections on learning. In: AAAI, vol. 4, p. 12 (2017)
16. Huang, G., Liu, Z., Van Der Maaten, L., et al.: Densely connected convolutional networks. In: CVPR, vol. 1, no. 2, p. 3 (2017)
17. Chollet, F.: Xception: deep learning with depthwise separable convolutions. arXiv preprint, 2017: 1610.02357 (2017)

Data Augmentation Based on Substituting Regional MRIs Volume Scores

Tuo Leng[1,2], Qingyu Zhao[2], Chao Yang[1], Zhufu Lu[1], Ehsan Adeli[2(✉)], and Kilian M. Pohl[2,3]

[1] School of Computer Engineering and Sciences, Shanghai University, Shanghai, China
eadeli@stanford.edu
[2] School of Medicine, Stanford University, Stanford, CA, USA
[3] SRI International, Center for Health Sciences, Menlo Park, CA, USA

Abstract. Due to difficulties in collecting sufficient training data, recent advances in neural-network-based methods have not been fully explored in the analysis of brain Magnetic Resonance Imaging (MRI). A possible solution to the limited-data issue is to augment the training set with synthetically generated data. In this paper, we propose a data augmentation strategy based on *regional feature substitution*. We demonstrate the advantages of this strategy with respect to training a simple neural-network-based classifier in predicting when individual youth transition from no-to-low to medium-to-heavy alcohol drinkers solely based on their volumetric MRI measurements. Based on 20-fold cross-validation, we generate more than one million synthetic samples from less than 500 subjects for each training run. The classifier achieves an accuracy of 74.1% in correctly distinguishing non-drinkers from drinkers at baseline and a 43.2% weighted accuracy in predicting the transition over a three year period (5-group classification task). Both accuracy scores are significantly better than training the classifier on the original dataset.

1 Introduction

In neuroimaging studies, structural Magnetic Resonance Imaging (MRI) is often used to examine the influence of neuropsychological diseases and disorders on brain structures [1–3]. These neuroscience studies frequently first extract morphometric measurements associated with regions-of-interest (ROI) from the brain MRI of each subject. Then statistical group analysis aims to identify disease-specific biomarkers by comparing these measurements between healthy and diseased subjects [4,5]. An alternative group analysis is to first train a classifier to accurately differentiate healthy subjects from diseased ones based on the measurements [6–8]. Then the subset of measurements highly influencing the classification outcome are identified as disease-specific imaging biomarkers.

The most advanced classification frameworks nowadays are arguably based on neural networks [7,8]. Despite their successful use in the computer vision

© Springer Nature Switzerland AG 2019
L. Zhou et al. (Eds.): LABELS 2019/HAL-MICCAI 2019/CuRIOUS 2019, LNCS 11851, pp. 32–41, 2019.
https://doi.org/10.1007/978-3-030-33642-4_4

community, it is well-known that the training of neural networks on medical imaging data suffers from the "high-dimension low-sample-size" problem [9]; that is, the number of subjects in each group is significantly lower than the dimension of measurements rendering the network easily overfitted. One way of alleviating this issue is to perform data augmentation, i.e., generating synthetic training data using information only from the existing training set, thereby reducing overfitting during training.

While affine transformations (including translation, flipping, and rotation) are commonly used for creating synthetic 3D MR images from existing ones [10], these operations are not meaningful for ROI-based measurements. Another commonly used augmentation strategy is based on adding Gaussian noise to the training data [10]. However, the noise level has to be manually chosen, which is not an intuitive procedure. For non-image data augmentation, approaches based on *feature-space warping* [11] have been proposed. These approaches aim to create synthetic data by warping the measurements of existing samples. For example, the Synthetic Minority Over-Sampling Technique (SMOTE) [12] computes the weighted average of measurements of two existing training subjects. Instead of synthesizing all measurements of a subject, we propose here a *regional-feature-substitution* strategy to incorporate the assumption commonly used in many neuroimaging studies [13] that brain morphometric measurements are only locally dependent and the fact that many neurological disorders only affect local brain regions [14]. Specifically, to create a new training sample, we substitute regional ROI measurements of an existing sample by those from another sample of the same cohort. We do so by arranging the ROI measurements as a matrix and substituting within sub-matrices, which we call "kernel" matrices. The kernel is constructed in compliance with the cortical parcellation of the brain to ensure that the warping only affects nearby brain regions.

In this study, we tested the augmentation strategy on the National Consortium on Alcohol and Neurodevelopment in Adolescence (NCANDA) dataset [15], which consists of longitudinal structural MRI scans of 505 subjects. The subjects were categorized into 5 groups according to their drinking behavior in the 4-year study period. We built a neural-network classifier to predict the group label based on the longitudinal measures of ROI cortical thickness. We show that by performing augmentation within each group separately to produce a well-balanced augmented dataset, our neural-network achieved a significant improvement on classification accuracy. Finally, we identify ROIs that highly influence the decision of the classifier through a visualization technique named layer-wise relevance propagation (LPR) [16].

2   Data Augmentation via Local Feature Warping

Suppose we have structural MRI images from S subjects that can be categorized into C groups. We further assume that morphometric measurements (e.g., gray-matter thickness) associated with V brain regions-of-interest (ROI) can be derived from each MRI image. We generalize the scenario to a longitudinal design, where these measurements are repeatedly measured T times, such that the measurements of each subject form a $T \times V$ matrix. Now, the V brain regions can be grouped into L major lobes, which we encode in the $T \times V$ matrix by arranging the columns so that neighboring ones are associated with ROIs belonging to the same lobe (see Fig. 1)

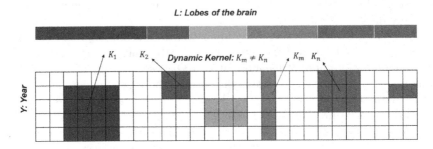

Fig. 1. Exemplar dynamic kernels within a toy measurement matrix. Columns are ordered such that ROIs of the same lobe (indicated by color) are adjacent. The location of a kernel is confined within a specific lobe.

To augment the training set, our approach is to "substitute" selective entries in the measurement matrices across subjects. To achieve this, we construct lobe-specific kernel matrices $K_l \in \mathbb{R}^{\alpha_l \times \beta_l}$, where $l \in \{1, 2, \cdots, L\}$ indicates the lobe and (α_l, β_l) indicates the size of the kernel. For instance, in the example of Fig. 1, $\alpha_1 = 4, \beta_1 = 4$ for K_1, and $\alpha_2 = 2, \beta_2 = 2$ for K_2. We then create a new synthetic subject by first randomly selecting a kernel and substituting the measurements inside the kernel of an existing subject by the ones from a different randomly-chosen subject in the same group (Fig. 2). As suggested by Fig. 1, the location of a kernel is confined within its specific lobe, so that the warping does not affect measurements of distant regions that are unlikely to correlate. Note that instead of using the weighted average strategy as in SMOTE that would generate unseen (thereby potentially unrealistic) measurements, our substitution strategy always uses existing measurements to synthesize new subjects.

Now let S_c denote the number of subjects in the cth group and V_l the number of ROIs in the lth lobe. Given the sizes $\{\alpha_l, \beta_l\}$ of the L kernels, the maximum number of subjects N that can be generated for a group is the product of the number of subject pairs (i.e., $(S_c - 1) \cdot S_c$) and the number of possible kernel matrices in all lobes:

$$N := \sum_{c=1}^{C} S_c (S_c - 1) \sum_{l=1}^{L} (T - \alpha_l + 1)(V_l - \beta_l + 1) \qquad (1)$$

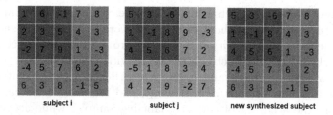

Fig. 2. Measurements of subject i within the kernel (blue) are substituted by the ones of subject j (green) to yield the measurements a new synthetic subject. (Color figure online)

3 Experimental Setup

3.1 Dataset

The experiments were based on data from the NCANDA study [15] comprised of 4-visit longitudinal data of 505 adolescents ($S = 505$, ages 12–22, 250 boys/255 girls; the data release NCANDA_PUBLIC_Y3_STRUCTURAL_V01 is made public according to the NCANDA Data Distribution agreement[1]). Each subject had 4 T1-weighted MRI scans ($T = 4$) that were acquired annually. They were categorized into 5 groups according to the specific year the subject transitioned from a no-to-low to medium-to-heavy alcohol drinker [15]. As shown in our previous studies [17], initiation of binge drinking alters normal development of brain morphometric patterns, so we hypothesize that subjects from different groups can be classified based on their brain morphometric measurements. In doing so, we have $S_1 = 265$ subjects who met the no-to-low drinking criteria of the NCANDA study [15] at baseline and throughout the study, $S_2 = 49$ subjects who met the criteria for the first 3 visits but transitioned to exceed-criteria drinkers at visit 4, $S_3 = 56$ transitioned at visit 3, $S_4 = 58$ transitioned at visit 2, $S_5 = 77$ subjects who remained exceeds-criteria drinkers throughout the study. Structural MRIs were processed using the publicly available NCANDA pipeline [17]. FreeSurfer (V 5.3.0) was applied to the skull-stripped MR images yielding the measurements of average thickness associated with 34 bilateral cortical ROIs ($V = 34$). Then confounders including age, sex, race and supratentorial volume were removed from the raw thickness measurements by general linear model analysis [14], which resulted in a 4×34 residual score matrix for each subject. Based on these score matrices, our goal was to apply data augmentation to train a classifier that could accurately predict the group label of each subject.

3.2 Data Augmentation for Classification

We tested whether the proposed data augmentation strategy could boost classification accuracy in two scenarios: 5-group classification and binary classification

---

[1] https://www.niaaa.nih.gov/research/major-initiatives/national-consortium-alcohol-and-neurodevelopment-adolescence.

between Group 1 and 5 (subjects remained non-heavy or heavy drinking through the 4-year study period) as these two groups were most distinguishable with respect to their drinking history across the 5 groups. For either scenario, the accuracy of classifiers in correctly labelling individuals was derived based on a 20-fold cross validation. The training data was enriched with the synthetic samples produced by our augmentation strategy, and the normalized classification accuracy (i.e., the accuracy of correctly labeling samples while accounting for differences in sample size among groups) was measured on the testing fold. Next, we detail the setup of kernel matrices used in our augmentation strategy and describe the up-sampling strategy as a benchmark approach in our experiments.

Table 1. Kernel dimension setup of 5-group (upper) and binary (lower) classification

Group	Temporal	Frontal	Occipital	Parietal	Cingulate	Insula
1	(4,9)	(4,11)	(4,4)	(4,5)	(4,4)	(4,1)
2	(1,1)	(1,1)	(1,1)	(1,1)	(1,1)	(1,1)
3	(1,4)	(1,1)	(1,1)	(1,1)	(1,1)	(1,1)
4	(1,5)	(1,1)	(1,1)	(1,1)	(1,1)	(1,1)
5	(1,8)	(2,6)	(2,1)	(2,1)	(2,1)	(2,1)
Group	Temporal	Frontal	Occipital	Parietal	Cingulate	Insula
1	(4,9)	(4,11)	(4,4)	(4,5)	(4,4)	(4,1)
2	(4,9)	(4,11)	(4,4)	(4,5)	(4,4)	(4,1)

Kernel Setup. Kernels were constructed with respect to the lobe parcellation of the brain. Adopting the Freesurfer parcellation, the brain was segmented into 6 major lobes: temporal lobe (9 ROIs), frontal lobe (11 ROIs), occipital lobe (4 ROIs), parietal lobe (5 ROIs), cingulate (4 ROIs) and insula. Given these dimensions, we set up kernel sizes ($\{\alpha_l, \beta_l\}$) such that the resulting augmented training set was as balanced as possible for the 5-group and binary classification (Table 1). Based on Eq. 1 and our kernel settings, the maximum number of synthetic samples generated from the training folds was 1,655,888, which was the sum of

$$
\begin{aligned}
N_1 &= 260 * (1 + 1 + 1 + 1 + 1 + 1) * 259 = 404040, \\
N_2 &= 44 * (36 + 44 + 16 + 20 + 16 + 4) * 43 = 257312, \\
N_3 &= 51 * (24 + 44 + 16 + 20 + 16 + 4) * 50 = 316200, \\
N_4 &= 53 * (20 + 44 + 16 + 20 + 16 + 4) * 52 = 330720, \\
N_5 &= 72 * (8 + 18 + 12 + 15 + 12 + 3) * 71 = 347616.
\end{aligned}
\tag{2}
$$

Similarly, the maximum size of augmentation for the binary classification task was $N = 344160 + 276060 = 620220$.

To relate the accuracy of classification with the size of the augmented training set, we also performed classification on subsets of the augmented dataset with different sizes (500, 2.5k, 50k, 250k, 500k). For each setting, the subset was randomly selected from the maximumly augmented training set while keeping the size of each group balanced.

Up-sampling. We also measured the classification accuracy when training was performed on balanced datasets generated by up-sampling (sample with replacement). Specifically, the raw training set was up-sampled to 2500 for 5-group and 430 for binary classification. Note that the size of these up-sampled datasets was determined to create a balanced training set rather than to perform data augmentation; Extensive up-sampling will only produce repeated training samples, so it does not improve the accuracy of the classifier.

3.3   Classifiers

The above data augmentation was independent of the choice of the classifier. Here, we tested the data-augmentation strategies on three different approaches: a simple, fully connected neural network called SmallNet as well as Random Forest (RF) and Supporting Vector Machine (SVM), two approaches that have been shown to be able to work reasonably on small training datasets. SmallNet only contained 3 hidden layers with each layer having 50 neurons. The activation function of each hidden layers was Relu, and the final output was the softmax functional for a general multi-group classification. To train our SmallNet classifier, the Kaiming's method [18] was used and initialized with a batch size of 128. Learning strategy of SmallNet was SGD with momentum of 0.1. All experiments were ran for 10 epochs at 0.0001 learning rate. During training, batch normalization and early stopping method were used for lowering the impact of overfitting. Note, we used SmallNet for simplification to illustrate the power of our augmentation strategy, and more sophisticated network structures might produce more accurate results. Our implementation of RF consisted of 100 decision trees. Each decision tree had the depth of up to 5, and the feature number for each split was 10. The weighted accuracy was obtained by averaging 100 training sessions. SVM was setup with a relaxation coefficient of 2.0, a maximum number of iterations of 5000, and an average of 50 out of 5000 cross-training. After 100 cross-training, the average was taken as the final results.

Table 2. Accuracy of 5-group and binary classification produced by random forest (RF), support vector machine (SVM) and SmallNet on different training sets.

Task	Training set	Size	RF	SVM	SmallNet
5-group classification	Raw data	405	19.9%	23.3%	19.2%
	Up-sampling	2500	27.5%	28.7%	23.1%
	Augmentation	1.6M	27.9%	29.3%	**44.1%**
Binary classification	Raw data	405	54.7%	57.7%	53.7%
	Up-sampling	430	55.6%	58.1%	56.1%
	Augmentation	600K	55.5%	58.2%	**73.8%**

4   Results

Here we analyze the accuracy of the 3 classifiers trained with and without data augmentation. We can see from Table 2 that all 3 classifiers performed poorly on the raw datasets for both 5-group and binary classification. When trained on the up-sampled dataset, the accuracy of RF and SVM slightly improved in the 5-group classification setting to approximately 28% (randomly labeling samples would produce an accuracy of 20%). However, these two methods showed little further improvement when the training set was augmented by the proposed strategy. On the other hand, even though SmallNet was often less accurate than RF and SVM on small training sets, it achieved significantly more accurate 5-group and binary classification results when trained on the augmented set. These results support the fact that RF and SVM are suitable for small to moderate datasets, so extensive data augmentation provides little merit. On the other hand, the implementation of neural networks requires a large-scale training dataset. In our specific application, training SmallNet benefited from the proposed data augmentation strategy resulting in the most accurate prediction for both classification settings. The above claims are further supported by Fig. 3. As the size of the augmented set increased, the accuracy of RF and SVM only increased marginally, whereas SmallNet showed a significant improvement. The performance of SmallNet converged approximately at 250k training samples for 5-group and 50k for the binary classification task.

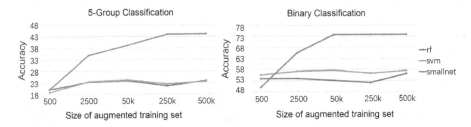

Fig. 3. Accuracy of RF, SVM and SmallNet based on different sizes of training dataset.

Visualization via LRP. As mentioned, another critical goal of most neuroimaging studies is to identify critical ROI biomarkers associated with specific cohorts, so we analyzed the subset of measurements that highly impacted the classification decision based on the Layer-wise relevance propagation (LRP) technique [16]. Given a feature matrix and a classifier, the aim of LRP is to assign each entry of the measurement matrix a relevance score such that negative scores contain evidence against the presence of a class, while positive scores contain evidence for the presence of a class. These pixel-wise relevance scores can be visualized as an image called *heatmap*. Here we focused the analysis on the binary classification as it highlighted the difference between normal adolescents (Group 1) and youth that had already initiated medium-to-heavy drinking at baseline (Group 5). Figure 4-left shows the heatmaps (relevance scores) associated with the input matrix. Yellow blocks in the upper figure correspond to the matrix entries that strongly indicate the presence of Group 1, whereas the yellow blocks below correspond to Group 5. The general agreement between the two heatmaps suggests that the binary classification was mainly based on several key measurements (in yellow). To relate those measurements to specific brain regions, these scores were averaged in the longitudinal dimension and then averaged between the two groups. The resulting 34-D vector was then color-coded on the cortical surface (Fig. 4 right). Yellow regions correspond to ROIs that contributed more to the prediction. We can see that brain regions in the temporal lobe (specifically superior temporal, fusiform, and inferior temporal regions) are more salient than others. The impact of alcoholism that leads to significant volume deficits in cortical gray/white matter in the temporal lobe has been frequently suggested in the alcohol literature [19].

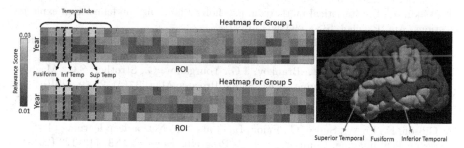

Fig. 4. Heat-map of relevance scores on the binary classification task

5   Conclusion

While data augmentation has been shown to be effective in increasing the performance of many image-based classifiers, our proposed augmentation strategy designed for ROI-measurements not only provided us sufficient data for training simple neural networks, but also showed a significant improvement on prediction results when applied to the NCANDA dataset. We showed that progression of drinking behaviors could be differentiated based on longitudinal brain morphometric measurements. Furthermore, by applying the LRP method, we were able to derive the relevance scores for the input measurement matrix, from which we could interpret and visualize the importance of ROIs in the decision process of the classifier.

In this work, however, we only explored kernel construction with respect to the spatial properties of the brain. We will further consider temporal correlation of the longitudinal measurements in constructing kernels. Moreover, we aim to extend the usage of our augmentation strategy in the context of image-based classification by applying regional warping to either raw images or intermediate features. This could potentially complement current image augmentation strategies based on global affine/deformable transformation.

Acknowledgement. This research was supported in part by NIH grants U24AA02 1697, AA005965, AA013521, AA026762, and National Natural Science Foundation of China grants 11501352, 61573235, 11871328.

References

1. Mueller, S., et al.: Ways toward an early diagnosis in Alzheimer's disease: the Alzheimer's disease neuroimaging initiative (ADNI). J. Alzheimers Dement. **1**(1), 55–66 (2005)
2. Frisoni, G.B., Fox, N.C., Jack, C.R., Scheltens, P., Thompson, P.M.: The clinical use of structural MRI in Alzheimer disease. Nat. Rev. Neurol. **6**(2), 67–77 (2011)
3. Di Martino, A., Yan, C.G., Li, Q., et al.: The autism brain imaging data exchange: towards a large-scale evaluation of the intrinsic brain architecture in autism. Mol. Psychiatry **19**(6), 659–667 (2014)
4. Wilkinson, L.: Statistical methods in psychology journals; guidelines and explanations. Am. Psychol. **5**(8), 594–604 (1999)
5. Madsen, H., Thyregod, P.: Introduction to General and Generalized Linear Models. Chapman & Hall/CRC, Boca Raton (2011)
6. Wernick, M.N., Yang, Y., Brankov, J.G., Yourganov, G., Strother, S.C.: Machine learning in medical imaging. IEEE Signal Process. Mag. **27**(4), 25–38 (2010)
7. Shen, D., Wu, G., Suk, H.I.: Deep learning in medical image analysis. Annu. Rev. Biomed. Eng. **19**, 221–248 (2017)
8. Gibson, E., Li, W., Sudre, C., Fidon, L., et al.: NiftyNet: a deep-learning platform for medical imaging. Comput. Methods Programs Biomed. **158**, 113–122 (2018)
9. Tajbakhsh, N., et al.: Convolutional neural networks for medical image analysis: Full training or fine tuning? IEEE TMI **35**(5), 1299–1312 (2016)
10. Hussain, Z., Gimenez, F., Yi, D., Rubin, D.: Differential data augmentation techniques for medical imaging classification tasks. In: AMIA Annual Symposium Proceedings, pp. 979–984 (2017)
11. Wong, S.C., Gatt, A., Stamatescu, V., McDonnell, M.D.: Understanding data augmentation for classification: when to warp? CoRR abs/1609.08764 (2016)
12. Chawla, N.V., Bowyer, K.W., Hall, L.O., Kegelmeyer, W.P.: SMOTE: synthetic minority over-sampling technique. J. Artif. Intell. Res. **16**, 321–357 (2002)
13. Bielza, C., Larranaga, P.: Bayesian networks in neuroscience: a survey. Front. Comput. Neurosci. **8**(131), 1–23 (2014)
14. Adeli, E., et al.: Chained regularization for identifying brain patterns specific to HIV infection. Neuroimage **183**, 425–437 (2018)
15. Brown, S., Brumback, T., Tomlinson, K., et al.: The national consortium on alcohol and neurodevelopment in adolescence (NCANDA): a multisite study of adolescent development and substance use. J. Stud. Alcohol Drugs **76**(6), 895–908 (2015)
16. Bach, S., Binder, A., Montavon, G., Klauschen, F., Müller, K.R., Samek, W.: On pixel-wise explanations for non-linear classifier decisions by layer-wise relevance propagation. PLoS ONE **10**(7), 1–46 (2015)
17. Pfefferbaum, A., Kwon, D., Brumback, T., et al.: Altered brain developmental trajectories in adolescents after initiating drinking. Am. J. Psychiatry **175**(4), 370–380 (2018)

18. He, K., Zhang, X., Ren, S., Sun, J.: Delving deep into rectifiers: surpassing human-level performance on ImageNet classification. In: The IEEE International Conference on Computer Vision (ICCV) (2015)
19. Pfefferbaum, A., et al.: Brain gray and white matter volume loss accelerates with aging in chronic alcoholics: a quantitative mri study. Alcohol. Clin. Exp. Res. **16**(6), 1078–1089 (1992)

Weakly Supervised Segmentation from Extreme Points

Holger Roth[✉], Ling Zhang, Dong Yang, Fausto Milletari, Ziyue Xu,
Xiaosong Wang, and Daguang Xu

NVIDIA, Bethesda, USA
{hroth,lingz,dongy,fmilletari,ziyuex,xiaosongw,daguangx}@nvidia.com

Abstract. Annotation of medical images has been a major bottleneck
for the development of accurate and robust machine learning models.
Annotation is costly and time-consuming and typically requires expert
knowledge, especially in the medical domain. Here, we propose to use
minimal user interaction in the form of extreme point clicks in order to
train a segmentation model that can, in turn, be used to speed up the
annotation of medical images. We use extreme points in each dimension
of a 3D medical image to constrain an initial segmentation based on
the random walker algorithm. This segmentation is then used as a weak
supervisory signal to train a fully convolutional network that can segment
the organ of interest based on the provided user clicks. We show that the
network's predictions can be refined through several iterations of training
and prediction using the same weakly annotated data. Ultimately, our
method has the potential to speed up the generation process of new
training datasets for the development of new machine learning and deep
learning-based models for, but not exclusively, medical image analysis.

1 Introduction

The growing number of medical images taken in routine clinical practice increases
the demand for machine learning (ML) methods to improve image analysis workflows. However, a major bottleneck for the development of novel ML-based models to integrate and increase the productivity of clinical workflows is the annotation of datasets that are useful to train such models. At the same time, volumetric analysis has shown several advantages over 2D measurements for clinical
applications [1], which further increases the amount of data (a typical CT scan
contains hundreds of slices) needing to be annotated in order to train accurate
3D models. However, the majority of annotation tools available today for medical imaging are constrained to annotation in multiplanar reformatted views.
The annotator needs to either brush paint or draw boundaries around organs of
interest, often on a slice-by-slice basis. Classical techniques like 3D region growing or interpolation tools can speed up the annotation process by starting from
seed points or allowing the user to skip certain slices. However, their usability is
often limited to certain types of structures and might not work well in general.

© Springer Nature Switzerland AG 2019
L. Zhou et al. (Eds.): LABELS 2019/HAL-MICCAI 2019/CuRIOUS 2019, LNCS 11851, pp. 42–50, 2019.
https://doi.org/10.1007/978-3-030-33642-4_5

Here, we propose to use minimal user interaction in form of extreme point clicks, together with iterative training and refinement. Starting from user-defined extreme points in each dimension of a 3D medical image, an initial segmentation is produced based on the random walker algorithm. This segmentation is then used as a weak supervisory signal to train a fully convolutional network that can segment the organ of interest based on the provided user clicks. We show that the network's predictions can be iteratively refined by using several iterations of training and prediction using the same weakly annotated data.

Related Work: Fully convolutional networks (FCNs) [2] have established themselves as the state-of-the-art methods for medical image segmentation in recent years [3–5]. However, a major drawback is that they are very data hungry, limiting their application in healthcare where data annotation is very expensive. In order to reduce the cost of labeling, semi-automated/interactive and weakly supervised methods have been proposed in the literature.

Building on recent advances in deep learning (DL), several methods have been proposed to integrate it with interactive segmentation schemes. DL has been used in [6] for the DeepIGeoS algorithms, which leverages geodesic distance transforms and user scribbles to allow interactive segmentation. Such a method does not exhibit robust performance when seeking segmentation for unseen object classes. An alternative method [7] uses image-specific fine-tuning and leveraging both bounding boxes and scribble-based interaction. In [8], the authors utilize point clicks that are modeled as Gaussian kernels in a separate input channel to a segmentation FCN in order to model user interactions via seed-point placing. Finally [9] proposes to use user-provided scribbles with random walks [10] and FCN predictions to achieve semi-automated segmentation of cardiac CT images. This method differs from our proposed method in that we only expect the user to provide extreme points rather than scribbles as initial input to the random walker algorithm and uses a different approach when iteratively refining the segmentations.

One of the first approaches using bounding box based weakly supervised training of deep neural networks in medical imaging was by [11]. They used a patch-based classification CNN to segment brain and lung regions using an initial *GrabCut* segmentation. After several rounds of predictions using CNN plus Dense CRF post-processing, the network's segmentation performance could be improved. Weakly-supervised or self-learning in medical image analysis can also make use of measurements readily available in the hospital picture archiving and communication system (PACS) such as measurements acquired during evaluation of the RECIST criteria [12]. However, these measurements are typically constraint to 2D and might miss adequate constraints for more complex three-dimensional shapes. In [13], unsupervised segmentation results are used to train a deep segmentation network on cystic lung regions, again in a slice-by-slice fashion. This approach might work well for certain organs, like the lungs, where an unsupervised technique can have good enough initial performance due to the good image contrast. However, completely unsupervised techniques might fail to generalize to organs where the boundary information is not as clear.

More recently, [14] introduced inequality constraints based on target-region size and image tags in the loss function of a CNN in order to train the network for weakly supervised segmentation.

2 Method

In this work, we approach initial interactive segmentation using user-provided clicks on the extreme points of the organ of interest. The overall proposed algorithm for weakly supervised segmentation from extreme points can be divided into the following steps which are detailed below:

1. Extreme point selection
2. Initial segmentation from scribbles via random walker algorithm
3. Segmentation via deep fully convolutional network
4. Regularization using random walker algorithm

Steps 2, 3, and 4 will be iterated until convergence. Here, convergence is defined based on the differences between two consecutive rounds of predictions as in [13].

1. Extreme point selection: Defining extreme points on the organ surface will allow the extraction of a bounding box around the organ (plus some padding $p = 20$ mm in all our experiment). Bounding box selection significantly reduces the image content that the 3D FCN has to analyze and simplifies the machine learning problem, as previous work on cascaded approaches has shown [15]. Bounding boxes and extreme points on objects have been widely studied in the computer vision literature [16]. Bounding boxes have a practical disadvantage in that the user often has to select the corners of bounding boxes that lie outside the object of interest. This is especially tricky to do for three-dimensional objects where the user typically has to navigate three multi-planar reformatted views (axial, coronal, sagittal) in order to achieve the task. Recent studies have also shown the time savings using extreme point selection brings for 2D object selection instead of traditional bounding box selection [16,17]. At the same time, extreme points provide additional information to the segmentation model (which can be observed in our experimental section, Table 1. They lie on the object surface and we model them as an additional input channel together with the image intensities. This extra channel includes 3D Gaussians G centered on each point location clicked by the user. This approach is similar to [16] but here we extended it to 3D medical imaging problems.

Figure 1 illustrates our approach. We ask the user to click on six extreme points (here four are shown in axial view) that describe the largest extent of the organ. These points are then used to compute a bounding box B automatically, including some padding p.

2. Initial segmentation from scribbles via random walker algorithm: In order to make use of extreme point clicks as a weak supervision signal, we turn them into a probability map $\hat{Y}$ than can act as a pseudo dense label map for driving a 3D FCN to learn the segmentation task. Based on the initial set

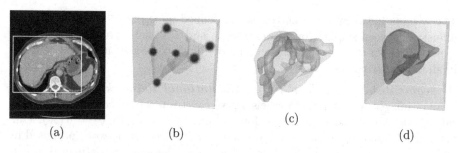

(a)   (b)   (d)

Fig. 1. Our weakly supervised segmentation framework. (a) The user selects extreme points that define the organ of interest (here the liver) in 3D space. (b) Extreme points are modeled as Gaussians in an extra image channel which is fed to a 3D segmentation model. (c) Foreground scribbles are generated automatically to initialize random walker (the ground truth surface is shown in red for reference). (d) Model returns the segmentation results.

of extreme points, we compute a set of foreground and background scribbles that act as the input seeds for the random walker algorithm [10]. We compute Dijkstra's shortest path [18] between each extreme point pair along each image dimension, where we model the distance between neighboring voxels by their gradient magnitude $D = \sqrt{\left(\frac{\partial f}{\partial x}\right)^2 + \left(\frac{\partial f}{\partial y}\right)^2 + \left(\frac{\partial f}{\partial z}\right)^2}$. Here, the shortest path result can be seen as an approximation of the geodesic distance [6] between the two extreme points in each dimension. Figure 1 shows the foreground scribbles used as input seeds to the random walker algorithm. In order to increase the number of foreground seeds, each path is also dilated with a 3D ball structure element of $r_{\text{foreground}} = 2$. The background seeds are defined as the dilated and inverted version of the input scribbles. While the amount of dilation does depend on the size of the organ of interest, we typically dilate with a ball structure element of radius $r_{\text{background}} = 30$ which achieves good initial seeds for organs like spleen, and liver.

Next, the random walker algorithm [10] is used to generate an initial prediction map $\hat{Y}$ based on the background s_0 and foreground s_1 scribbles described above. The random walker basically solves the diffusion equation between voxels defined as source and sink as defined by the scribbles S. Here, the 3D volume is defined as a graph $G(E, V)$ with edges $e \in E$ and vertices $v \in V$. The edge between two vertices v_i and v_j is denoted as e_{ij} and can be assigned a weight w_{ij} based on the image intensities gradients. Furthermore, the degree of a given vertex is defined by $d_i = \sum w_{ij}$. We solve the diffusion equation in order to get a probability $p(\omega|x) = x_j^\omega$ for each vertex v_i to belong to the foreground class ω_1. Here, L is the Laplacian of the weighted image graph G with each element of the matrix defined as:

$$L_{ij} = \begin{cases} d_i, & \text{if } i = j, \\ -w_{ij}, & \text{if } i \text{ and } j \text{ are adjacent voxels,} \\ 0, & \text{otherwise} \end{cases} \qquad (1)$$

The weights between adjacent voxels are defined as $w_{ij} = e^{-\beta|z_j-z_i|^2}$ to make diffusion between similar voxel intensities z_i and z_j easier. While β is a tunable hyperparameter that controls the amount of diffusion, we keep it fixed at $\beta = 130$ in all our experiments.

3. Segmentation via deep fully convolutional network: Next, given all pairs of images X and pseudo labels $\hat{Y}$, we can train a fully convolutional neural network to segment the given foreground class, with $P(X) = f(X)$. Our network architecture of choice follows the encoder-decoder network proposed in [19], utilizing an-isotropic $(3 \times 3 \times 1)$ kernels in the encoder path in order to make use of pretrained weights from 2D computer vision tasks. As in [19], we initialize from *ImageNet* pretrained weights using a ResNet-18 encoder branch. While the initial weights are learned from 2D, all convolutions are still applied in a full 3D fashion throughout the network, allowing it to efficiently learn 3D features from the image. The Dice loss [4] has been established as the objective function of choice for medical image segmentation tasks. Its properties allow automatic scaling to unbalanced labeling problems. At the same time, it also naturally adapts to the comparing probability maps without any modifications to the original formulation:

$$\mathcal{L}_{Dice} = 1 - \frac{2 \sum_{i=1}^{N} y_i \hat{y}_i}{\sum_{i=1}^{N} y_i^2 + \sum_{i=1}^{N} \hat{y}_i^2} \tag{2}$$

Here, y_i is the predicted probability from our network f and $\hat{y}_i$ is the weak label probability from our pseudo label map $\hat{Y}$ at voxel i.

4. Regularization using random walker algorithm: We could stop our learning after the segmentation network f above is trained on the pseudo labels $\hat{Y}$. However, we notice that an additional regularization step by an additional random walker segmentation as described above can be very beneficial to the convergence of our weakly-supervised segmentation approach. This finding is similar in spirit to [11], where a DenseCRF is utilized after each round of CNN training in order to introduce regularization to the segmentation output. In order to increase the amount of regularization the random walker can bring to the network's predictions, we add an area of uncertainty by eroding the foreground prediction $P(X) >= 0.5$ and eroding the background $P(X) < 0.5$ both with a ball structure element of radius $r_{randomwalker} = 4$ in all our experiments. This allows the random walker to produce new predictions around the boundary of the foreground object that differ from the previous 3D FCN predictions and in turn, help the next iteration to learn new features from the same set of training images, and not to get stuck in a local optimum. In fact, we notice that without this step, our weakly supervised segmentation framework becomes unstable and does not easily converge to a satisfying performance.

3   Experiments and Results

Datasets: We utilize the training datasets (as they include ground truth annotations) from public challenges, specifically, from the *Medical Segmentation*

Decathlon[1] and the *Challenge on Endocardial Three-dimensional Ultrasound Segmentation*[2]. All numbers are reported on 1 mm isotropic images that were generated from the original images using linear interpolation for both CT and MRI images. For ultrasound images, we keep their original resolution as they are close to isotropic. We employ random splits for training and validation for all datasets, resulting 32/9 cases for spleen (CT), 104/27 cases for liver (CT), 26/6 cases for prostate (MRI), and 24/6 cases for left ventricle (LV) in ultrasound (US).

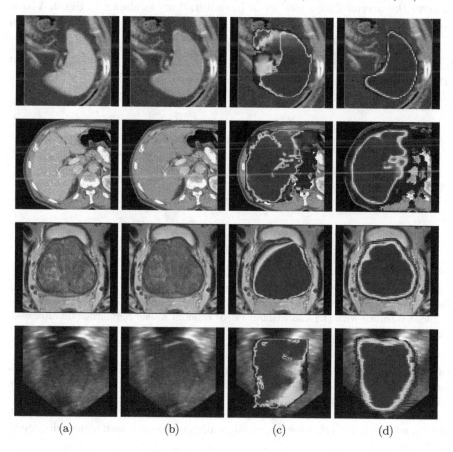

(a)   (b)   (c)   (d)

Fig. 2. Our results. We show (a) the image, (b) overlaid (full) ground truth (used for evaluation only), (c) initial random walker prediction, and (d) our final segmentation result produced by the weakly supervised FCN. We show qualitative results for top to bottom: spleen (CT), liver (CT), prostate (MRI), and left ventricle (US) segmentation.

Experiments: In all cases, we iterate our algorithm until convergence on the validation data. We compare both training with and without employing random walker (RW) regularization after each round of 3D FCN training. Furthermore,

---

[1] http://medicaldecathlon.com.

[2] https://www.creatis.insa-lyon.fr/Challenge/CETUS/.

we quantify the benefit of modelling the extreme points as an extra input channel to the network by running the framework with RW regularization but without the extreme points channel. The results are summarized in Table 1 for all segmentation tasks. It can be observed that the biggest improvements happen in the first round FCN learning after initial random walker segmentation. While random walker regularization does not always improve the average Dice score, it does help to introduce enough "novelty" into our learning framework in order to drive the overall Dice score up in later iterations as shown in Fig. 3. Visual examples of the improvement between from initial random walker to the final FCN prediction is shown in Fig. 2.

Implementation: The training and evaluation of the deep neural networks used in the proposed framework were implemented based on the *NVIDIA Clara Train SDK*[3] using NVIDIA Tesla V100 GPUs with 16 GB memory.

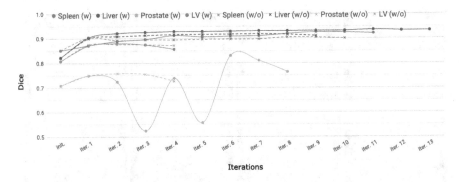

Fig. 3. Weakly supervised training from scribble based initialization. Each segmentation task is shown with (w) and without (w/o) random walker regularization after each round of FCN training.

Table 1. Summary of our weakly supervised segmentation results. This table compares the random walker initialization with weakly supervised training from extreme points with (w) and without (w/o) random walker (RW) regularization, and with RW regularization but without the extra extreme points channel as input to the network (w RW; no extr.). For reference, the performance on the same task under fully supervised training is shown.

Dice	Spleen (CT)	Liver (CT)	Prostate (MRI)	LV (US)
Rnd. walk. init.	0.852	0.822	0.709	0.808
Weak. sup. (w/o RW)	0.905	0.918	0.758	0.876
Weak. sup. (w RW; no extr.)	0.924	0.935	0.779	0.860
Weak. sup. (w RW)	**0.926**	**0.936**	**0.830**	**0.880**
Fully supervised	*0.963*	*0.958*	*0.923*	*0.903*

---

[3] https://devblogs.nvidia.com/annotate-adapt-model-medical-imaging-clara-train-sdk.

4   Discussion and Conclusions

We presented a method for weakly supervised 3D segmentation from extreme points. Asking the user to select the organ of interest using simple point clicks on the organ's surface in each spatial dimension can reduce the amount of labeling cost drastically. At the same time, the point clicks can describe the region of interest and simplify the machine learning task in 3D. Furthermore, the extreme points can be utilized to generate an initial weak pseudo label based on the extreme points utilizing the random walker algorithm. We found our initial label to be relatively robust to three diverse medical image segmentation tasks involving three different image modalities (CT, MRI, and ultrasound). Occasionally, the random walker can lack robustness for organs showing very diverse interior textures, like some advanced cancer patients in the prostate dataset. Here, a boundary search algorithm could potentially provide a better initial segmentation. Still, our FCN training in is able to markedly improve upon the initial segmentation. Previous work mainly utilized bounding box annotations for weakly supervised learning, e.g. [11]. However, we consider selecting extreme points on the organ's surface to be more natural then selecting corners of a bounding box outside the organ of interest and more efficient than adding scribbles inside and around the organ [6,9]. This is consistent to findings in the computer vision literature [17]. In the future, the region of interest and extreme point selection could be replaced by an automatic proposal network in order to further reduce the manual burden of medical image annotation.

References

1. Devaraj, A., van Ginneken, B., Nair, A., Baldwin, D.: Use of volumetry for lung nodule management: theory and practice. Radiology **284**(3), 630–644 (2017)
2. Long, J., Shelhamer, E., Darrell, T.: Fully convolutional networks for semantic segmentation. In: CVPR, 3431–3440 (2015)
3. Ronneberger, O., Fischer, P., Brox, T.: U-Net: convolutional networks for biomedical image segmentation. In: Navab, N., Hornegger, J., Wells, W.M., Frangi, A.F. (eds.) MICCAI 2015. LNCS, vol. 9351, pp. 234–241. Springer, Cham (2015). https://doi.org/10.1007/978-3-319-24574-4_28
4. Milletari, F., Navab, N., Ahmadi, S.A.: V-Net: fully convolutional neural networks for volumetric medical image segmentation. In: 3D Vision, pp. 565–571. IEEE (2016)
5. Çiçek, Ö., Abdulkadir, A., Lienkamp, S.S., Brox, T., Ronneberger, O.: 3D U-Net: learning dense volumetric segmentation from sparse annotation. In: Ourselin, S., Joskowicz, L., Sabuncu, M.R., Unal, G., Wells, W. (eds.) MICCAI 2016. LNCS, vol. 9901, pp. 424–432. Springer, Cham (2016). https://doi.org/10.1007/978-3-319-46723-8_49
6. Wang, G., et al.: DeepIGeoS: a deep interactive geodesic framework for medical image segmentation. IEEE Trans. Pattern Anal. Mach. Intell. **41**, 1559–1572 (2018)
7. Wang, G., et al.: Interactive medical image segmentation using deep learning with image-specific fine tuning. IEEE Trans. Med. Imaging **37**(7), 1562–1573 (2018)

8. Sakinis, T., et al.: Interactive segmentation of medical images through fully convolutional neural networks. arXiv preprint arXiv:1903.08205 (2019)
9. Can, Y.B., Chaitanya, K., Mustafa, B., Koch, L.M., Konukoglu, E., Baumgartner, C.F.: Learning to segment medical images with scribble-supervision alone. In: Stoyanov, D., et al. (eds.) DLMIA/ML-CDS -2018. LNCS, vol. 11045, pp. 236–244. Springer, Cham (2018). https://doi.org/10.1007/978-3-030-00889-5_27
10. Grady, L.: Random walks for image segmentation. IEEE Trans. Pattern Anal. Mach. Intell. 1768–1783(11) (2006)
11. Rajchl, M., et al.: DeepCut: object segmentation from bounding box annotations using convolutional neural networks. IEEE Trans. Med. Imaging **36**(2), 674–683 (2017)
12. Cai, J., et al.: Accurate weakly supervised deep lesion segmentation on CT scans: Self-paced 3D mask generation from RECIST. arXiv preprint arXiv:1801.08614 (2018)
13. Zhang, L., Gopalakrishnan, V., Lu, L., Summers, R.M., Moss, J., Yao, J.: Self-learning to detect and segment cysts in lung ct images without manual annotation. In: ISBI, pp. 1100–1103. IEEE (2018)
14. Kervadec, H., Dolz, J., Tang, M., Granger, E., Boykov, Y., Ayed, I.B.: Constrained-CNN losses for weakly supervised segmentation. Med. Image Anal. **54**, 88–99 (2019)
15. Roth, H.R., et al.: Spatial aggregation of holistically-nested convolutional neural networks for automated pancreas localization and segmentation. Med. Image Anal. **45**, 94–107 (2018)
16. Maninis, K.K., Caelles, S., Pont-Tuset, J., Van Gool, L.: Deep extreme cut: From extreme points to object segmentation. In: CVPR, pp. 616–625 (2018)
17. Papadopoulos, D.P., Uijlings, J.R., Keller, F., Ferrari, V.: Extreme clicking for efficient object annotation. In: ICCV, pp. 4930–4939 (2017)
18. Dijkstra, E.W.: A note on two problems in connexion with graphs. Numerische mathematik **1**(1), 269–271 (1959)
19. Liu, S., et al.: 3D anisotropic hybrid network: transferring convolutional features from 2D images to 3D anisotropic volumes. In: Frangi, A.F., Schnabel, J.A., Davatzikos, C., Alberola-López, C., Fichtinger, G. (eds.) MICCAI 2018. LNCS, vol. 11071, pp. 851–858. Springer, Cham (2018). https://doi.org/10.1007/978-3-030-00934-2_94

Exploring the Relationship Between Segmentation Uncertainty, Segmentation Performance and Inter-observer Variability with Probabilistic Networks

Elisa Chotzoglou$^{(\boxtimes)}$ and Bernhard Kainz

Department of Computing, BioMedIA, Imperial College London, London, UK
{e.chotzoglou16,b.kainz}@imperial.ac.uk

Abstract. Medical image segmentation is an essential tool for clinical decision making and treatment planning. Automation of this process led to significant improvements in diagnostics and patient care, especially after recent breakthroughs that have been triggered by deep learning. However, when integrating automatic tools into patient care, it is crucial to understand their limitations and to have means to assess their confidence for individual cases. Aleatoric and epistemic uncertainties have been subject of recent research. Methods have been developed to calculate these quantities automatically during segmentation inference. However, it is still unclear how much human factors affect these metrics. Varying image quality and different levels of human annotator expertise are an integral part of aleatoric uncertainty. It is unknown how much this variability affects uncertainty in the final segmentation. Thus, in this work we explore potential links between deep network segmentation uncertainties with inter-observer variance and segmentation performance. We show how the area of disagreement between different ground-truth annotators can be developed into model confidence metrics and evaluate them on the LIDC-IDRI dataset, which contains multiple expert annotations for each subject. Our results indicate that a probabilistic 3D U-Net and a 3D U-Net using Monte-Carlo dropout during inference both show a similar correlation between our segmentation uncertainty metrics, segmentation performance and human expert variability.

1 Introduction

Segmentation, *i.e.*, delineation of anatomical structures in 2D/3D, is a core necessity in medical imaging analysis. In most cases, segmentation is carried out manually by an expert. It is well known that manual segmentation suffers from inter-observer variability and that segmentation quality is influenced by factors such as fatigue, different domain knowledge, level of expertise, and image resolution. As a result, manual segmentations contain aleatoric uncertainty and can thus be ambiguous for diagnosis or confusing for supervised learning methods. Nevertheless, annotator confidence can be an important source of information for

© Springer Nature Switzerland AG 2019
L. Zhou et al. (Eds.): LABELS 2019/HAL-MICCAI 2019/CuRIOUS 2019, LNCS 11851, pp. 51–60, 2019.
https://doi.org/10.1007/978-3-030-33642-4_6

clinical decision making. Varying annotator confidence can be a trigger for additional imaging tests and an indicator for quality control and treatment options. Confidence is an important factor to weigh individual test result but it is only qualitatively assessed in the clinical practice. Recent successes of deep learning for image segmentation [2,8] promise to reduce clinical annotation workload. Currently, the majority of these methods lack the ability to communicate annotator confidence.

Quantitative assessment of uncertainties is key to guarantee quality of care, increases trust and can have great impact on therapeutic decisions. Thus, in this work we explore whether human inter-observer variability can be correlated with the distribution of two different probabilistic neural networks and investigate the impact of this variability on the estimation of segmentation uncertainty and segmentation performance. To achieve this, we

(1) discuss an extension of a probabilistic U-Net [10] to 3D,
(2) compare the properties of a 3D probabilistic U-Net with a Monte-Carlo dropout extension of a standard 3D U-Net [2] on the proof-of-concept task of lung nodule segmentation,
(3) examine and present both qualitatively and quantitatively at which extent automatically predicted confidence and uncertainty metrics, disagreement aware metric (which is proposed) and segmentation performance metrics are correlated.

Related Work: Estimation of uncertainty in the medical imaging domain has been attempted in works such as [11,12,14]. In [14] authors use Monte Carlo samples from the posterior distribution of a Bayesian fully Convolutional neural network which are derived using dropout at test phase. Based on these samples, they compute structure-wise and voxel-wise uncertainties metrics, which as they prove, are highly correlated with segmentation accuracy. Application field is infant brain segmentation. In another work [12] Monte Carlo dropout is used for uncertainty estimation in Multiple Sclerosis lesion detection and segmentation. Four different voxel-wise uncertainties were utilised including prediction variance, Monte Carlo sample variance, predictive Entropy and Mutual Information. As it was proved by the results, filtering based on uncertainty leads to improvement on the lesion detection accuracy. In [11] authors propose a framework to approximate Bayesian inference in deep neural networks by imposing Bernoulli distribution directly on the weights of the deep model. Then Monte Carlo samples from posterior distribution are utilised to compute Mutual Information as metric for uncertainty in CT-organ semantic segmentation. Furthermore, the effect of inter-observer variability for estimation of uncertainty in segmentation is studied in [7]. Authors, in MRI images from brain tumors, explore the impact of different label fusion techniques (e.g. no fusion, staples, union, intersection, majority) in estimation of segmentation uncertainty. As it is proved, there is a link between uncertainty estimation and inter-observer variability. Monte Carlo dropout is also used in this work for estimation of uncertainty (entropy). Finally, an alternative way to produce plausible segmentation hypotheses is proposed in [10] where authors use generative segmentation model, a combination of U-Net and conditional variational autoencoder, in order to produce plausible segmentation hypotheses (diverse samples) for lung abnormalities segmentation task.

2   Background

Two different probabilistic networks are utilised in our work: a $3D$ probabilistic U-Net (**PUNet**) and a $3D$ U-Net using Monte Carlo Dropout during inference (**DUNet**).

PUNet: We extend a $2D$ probabilistic U-Net [10], which is a combination of a U-Net [2,13] and a conditional variational autoencoder [17] to 3D. The whole architecture consists of three networks, which is shown in Fig. 1.

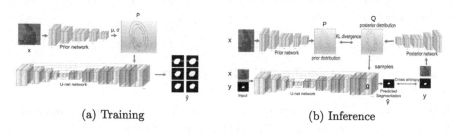

(a) Training   (b) Inference

Fig. 1. PUNet [10] as we use it for our method.

Let x be an input volume, M the segmentation map, $\hat{y}$ the predicted segmentation, y the ground truth segmentation as it is produced by several experts ($n = 4$ for LIDC), C the number of classes and N number of voxels per volume similar as proposed by [10]. The Prior net is conditioned on the input volume x. It computes the distribution over the (low-dimensional) latent space R^K. At inference stage samples that are produced by this distribution are concatenated with the last layer's feature maps of the segmentation network, which produces a segmentation map for each sample. More precisely the prior probability distribution P is modelled as an axis-aligned Gaussian distribution with mean $\mu_{prior}(x; w_{prior}) \in R^K$ and variance $\sigma_{prior}(x; w_{prior}) \in R^K$. To sample T segmentations we apply the network T times to the same input volume. In each iteration a sample $z_t, t = \{1, 2, ..., T\}$ is drawn from the distribution:

$$z \sim P(.|x) = \mathcal{N}(\mu_{prior}(x; w_{prior}), diag(\sigma_{prior}(x; w_{prior}))) \qquad (1)$$

Each sample is reshaped to a K-channel feature map with the same shape as the segmentation map. This feature map is concatenated to the last activation map of a U-Net. Then, a segmentation map, which corresponds to sample t, is produced by $M_t = f(g(x, w), z_i, \psi)$ where w is the U-Net parameters and ψ weights of the last layer of U-Net.

The posterior net is conditioned on the volume x as well as the ground truth y. It learns to recognize (embeds) segmentation variants $\mu_{post}(x, y; \nu) \in R^K$ with some uncertainty $\sigma_{post}(x, y; \nu) \in R^K$ in the low dimensional latent space. The output is denoted as posterior distribution Q. A sample z from this distribution

$$z \sim Q(.|x, y) = \mathcal{N}(\mu_{post}(x, y; \nu), diag(\sigma_{post}(x, y; \nu)) \qquad (2)$$

combined with the activation map of the U-Net will result in a predicted segmentation $\hat{y}$.

The loss function is composed by two terms. The first is the cross entropy loss $E_{z \sim Q(.|y, x)}[-\log P_c(y|M(x, z))]$, which penalizes the difference between the ground truth and the segmentation map. The second one is the Kullback-Leibler (KL) divergence $D_{KL}(Q(z|y, x)||P(z|x))$ which penalizes differences between the posterior distribution Q and the prior distribution P. Both terms are combined as a weighted sum with a weighting factor β as proposed by [10]. Thus, the total loss function is defined as:

$$L(y, x) = E_{z \sim Q(.|y, x)}[-\log P_c(y|M(x, z))] + \beta * D_{KL}(Q(z|y, x)||P(z|x)) \qquad (3)$$

In our experiments we use $\beta = 0.2$. Differences between training and inference are outlined in Fig. 1.

DUNet: We utilise a U-Net where dropout layers are activated during inference. During test phase, dropout is similar to Bayesian approximation [4]. In this way, we can take Monte Carlo samples over the posterior distribution $p(w|x, y)$ of the models' weight w and volume x and labels y. Cross entropy between ground truth and predicted segmentation is utilised as loss function.

3   Method

To produce plausible segmentation samples, we utilise PUNet and DUNet. In order to exploit volumetric information, $3D$ versions of the above models are trained using $3D$ convolutions. The U-Nets consist of 3 layers. Each layer consists of $3D$ convolution blocks followed by Rectified Linear Unit (ReLU) activation, batch normalization and max pooling. Filter size is $3 \times 3 \times 3$. We start the number of feature maps at 32 and double it after each block. For the prior net as well as for the posterior net in the PUNet, we utilize the encoder part of the U-Net. We train the networks using exponential decay learning rate and the Adam optimizer. For the DUNet, dropout is used after each layer in the encoding part of U-Net. We use a dropout probability of 0.2. We generate an equal number of samples T for both $3D$ networks. All networks are implemented in Python using Tensorflow, on a workstation with NVIDIA Titan X GPU.

In order to estimate model uncertainty we compute two uncertainty scores: Z_{var} and Z_S using variance [9,16] and predictive entropy [5] of samples respectively.

We define mean variance across all classes C as:

$$\sigma^2(x^*) = \frac{1}{C}\sum_{c=1}^{C}\frac{1}{T}\sum_{t=1}^{T}(p_t(y = c|x^*, w) - \hat{p}(y = c|x^*, w))^2, \tag{4}$$

where $\hat{p}(y|x^*, w)$ is the average of softmax probabilities of T samples for each $c \in [1, ..., C]$ and p_t the output of the network for sample t. Subsequently we define Z_{var} as

$$Z_{var} = \frac{1}{N}\sum_{v=1}^{N}\sigma^2(x^*(v)), \tag{5}$$

and predictive entropy S as

$$S(x^*) = -\sum_{c=1}^{C}\hat{p}(y = c|x^*, w) \times \log(\hat{p}(y = c|x^*, w)). \tag{6}$$

Thus, for each subject x^*, Z_S is computed as:

$$Z_S = \frac{1}{N}\sum_{v=1}^{N}S(x^*(v)) \tag{7}$$

We utilise the Sørensen–Dice coefficient (Dice score) to characterise segmentation performance. To examine possible linear correlation between segmentation performance and model uncertainty, we compute the Pearson correlation coefficient (ρ) between Z_S and Z_{var} and the Dice score.

To investigate the relationship between Z_S and Z_{var} and the variability among human experts we define the area of human disagreement (Γ) as an XOR ($\oplus$) of the different annotations for each subject. For each voxel the $\oplus$ operation will result 1 indicating that at least one annotator disagrees (disagreement) while 0 is used where all annotators agree (agreement). For a fair comparison with Z_S and Z_{var} we utilize the same schemes for deriving quantitative uncertainty: predictive Entropy(S) Eq. 6 and variance σ^2 Eq. 4. For qualitative analysis we imply Mutual Information (MI) and a map of softmax output probabilities for the predominant class (Softmax). MI is defined using Eq. 6 as the entropy of the average of samples minus the mean of the sum of the entropy of each sample, *i.e.*,

$$MI(x^*) = S(x^*) + \sum_{c=1}^{C}\frac{1}{T}\sum_{t=1}^{T}p_t(y = c|x^*, w)\log(p_t(y = c|x^*, w)), \tag{8}$$

where $p_t(y = c|x^*, w)$ is the softmax output of the network for each sample. We then characterise a voxel v of a new sample x^* as certain/uncertain using

$$x^*(v) = \begin{cases} \text{uncertain,} & \text{if } S(x^*(v)) >= \theta, \\ \text{certain,} & \text{otherwise,} \end{cases} \tag{9}$$

where θ is a threshold and v a voxel. Alternatively, we can replace $S(x^*)$ in Eq. 9 with variance σ^2 for estimation of uncertainty. We use a threshold since we assume that human perception of uncertainty is more accurate when interpreted binary than continuous. Evidence for this is given in behavioural sciences literature, *e.g.* [3,6].

We compute the ROC curve between True Positive Rate (TPR) and False Positive Rate (FPR) for the binary case. This allows us to correlate model uncertainty with aleatoric expert uncertainty. With Γ and Eq. 9 we define TPR and FPR as

$$\text{TPR} = p(\text{uncertain}|\text{disagreement}) = \frac{p(\text{uncertain, disagreement})}{p(\text{disagreement})}, \qquad (10)$$

and

$$\text{FPR} = p(\text{uncertain}|\text{agreement}) = \frac{p(\text{uncertain, agreement})}{p(\text{agreement})}. \qquad (11)$$

To evaluate segmentation uncertainty with respect to Γ we use disagreement accuracy (*DisAcc*) as metric [11,15]. *DisAcc* correlates positively with expert variability. It requires the definition of true invalid predictions, TI, as the voxels that are uncertain within in the area of disagreement (uncertain and disagreement) and true non-invalid prediciotns, TU, as the voxels that are certain in the area of agreement (certain and agreement). Similarly to conventional accuracy, *DisAcc* can be written as $DisAcc = \frac{TI+TU}{N}$, normalised by the total number of voxels N.

4   Evaluation and Results

Data. We use the LIDC-IDRI [1,18] dataset for training and testing. This CT dataset contains images of lung nodules and their delineations from four independent expert observers. We resample data to an isotropic volume resolution of $1 \times 1 \times 1 \text{ mm}^3$. We use 700 patients as a training dataset and 175 patients as a test set for performance evaluation. We crop each volume at the center of the nodule position and produce volumes of $128 \times 128 \times 128$. For the evaluation of the method we use the Dice score as a metric of volume overlap.

Correlation of Z_S and Z_{var} and Dice Score: We analyze correlation between Z_{var} and Z_S (Sect. 3) and the actual Dice score in Fig. 2. Dice score is computed between the absolute ground truth (average of 4 annotators) and the predicted segmentation. In Fig. 2(a, b, e, f) we observe linear negative correlation ($p < 0.001$) between Z_{var}, Z_S and the segmentation performance for both networks. Higher negative correlation is observed for DUNet between Z_{var} and Dice score (Fig. 2e, $\rho = -0.75$) and between Z_S and Dice score (Fig. 2f, $\rho = -0.67$).

There are some cases (10 cases) in both methods that produce uncertainty scores that are not representative for the segmentation quality. Although these nodules do not have any special visual characteristics, the model produces high Dice scores with high uncertainty scores. In Fig. 2c, d and g, h the distributions of uncertainty scores are plotted for two different groups of segmentations.

Successful segmentations have been empirically defined as those where the Dice score is ≥ 0.80 and unsuccessful segmentations with Dice scores ≤ 0.65. Thus, a threshold for the uncertainty score, which divides the two groups of segmentations can be defined as the intersection of the two distributions, which is close to 0.25.

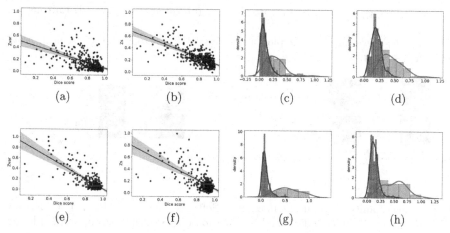

(a)   (b)   (c)   (d)

(e)   (f)   (g)   (h)

Fig. 2. Scatter plots of correlation between Dice score and uncertainty scores and probability density function (pdf) plots for both networks. Top row: PUNet. Bottom row: DUNet. Correlation between Dice score and Z_{var} and Z_S respectively: (a–b) PUNet and (e–f) for DUNet. Probability density function (PDF) for values of Z_{var} (and Z_S) of samples whose Dice scores is between 0.80 and 0.95 (blue) and the samples that their Dice scores is lower than 0.65 (red). (c–d) for PUNet and (g–h) for DUNet. (Color figure online)

Inter-observer Variability vs. Segmentation Uncertainty: As a naïve baseline we evaluate a convolutional regressor network to predict the annotator variance directly from the volumes. The regressor consists of 5 (convolution-max pooling) layers which are followed by a global average pooling (GAP) layer to predict $Z_{var} \in [0,1]$ directly. Mean square error between prediction and ground truth of variance among annotators is minimised during training. The performance of this approach is limited with a mean square error of 0.22 ± 0.0012. To evaluate TPR (Eq. 10) and FPR (Eq. 11) we compute ROC curves for each network as shown in Fig. 3 and evaluate *DisAcc* for a range of thresholds. The ROC curves of FPR and TPR (a–b) of both networks are quite similar with the best result for predictive entropy (Eq. 6) as uncertainty metric and PUNet with $AUC = 0.98$. Comparing *DisAcc* (c–d) for 5 different thresholds $\theta \in [0,1]$ for both networks and *DisAcc* reaches 0.99 for $\theta = 0.2$ and then remains stable.

Qualitative Analysis of Inter-observer Variability and Segmentation Uncertainty. Finally, we present a qualitative comparison between segmentation uncertainty and human uncertainty. Here, human uncertainty is expressed as human annotator entropy. We present and compare the result among all the different uncertainty metrics for both networks in Fig. 4.

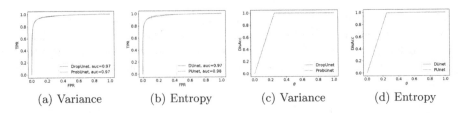

| (a) Variance | (b) Entropy | (c) Variance | (d) Entropy |

Fig. 3. ROC curves and *DisAcc* plots using predictive Entropy and σ^2 for both probabilistic networks

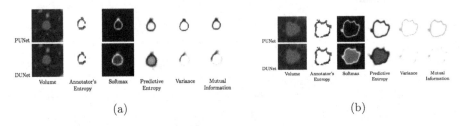

(a)   (b)

Fig. 4. Uncertainty maps using maximum Softmax ($\max(M)$), Predictive Entropy (Eq. 6), Variance (Eq. 4) and Mutual Information (Eq. 8) using both networks (darker colour, larger value).

5   Discussion

A limitation of our evaluation is that for a few cases the evaluated uncertainty scores are not a representative metric for how good or bad is a segmentation and it is likely dependant on the used data set. Furthermore, the impact of added parameter capacity in the probabilistic U-Net architecture compared to the dropout-only architecture will need to be carefully investigated in future work. Also, uncertainty as perceived by humans might be fundamentally different from model confidence. Although there is evidence that model uncertainty could capture/include also human disagreement area, it is not clear yet at which extend this happens. Finally, the impact of the different label fusion techniques in the estimation of ground truth and segmentation uncertainty will need to be further examined.

6   Conclusion

Using probabilistic 3D segmentation networks, we examine the relationship between segmentation uncertainty and segmentation performance. We explore to which extent human expert inter-observer variability can effect and correlate with model segmentation uncertainty. Our results show that both, a U-Net using MC dropout during inference as well as a 3D probabilistic U-Net architecture can quantitatively correlate the posterior segmentation distribution with true uncertainties. We present results that show a relationship between segmentation uncertainty and the area of annotator disagreement. Thus, in most cases model segmentation uncertainty indicates also likely human disagreement. The integration of the evaluated metrics into clinical quality control or for example into an active learning framework, where 'uncertain' parts of segmentations will be re-processed by a human, might show benefit in future work.

References

1. Armato III, S.G., et al.: The lung image database consortium (LIDC) and image database resource initiative (IDRI): a completed reference database of lung nodules on CT scans. Med. Phys. **38**(2), 915–931 (2011)
2. Çiçek, Ö., Abdulkadir, A., Lienkamp, S.S., Brox, T., Ronneberger, O.: 3D U-Net: learning dense volumetric segmentation from sparse annotation. In: Ourselin, S., Joskowicz, L., Sabuncu, M.R., Unal, G., Wells, W. (eds.) MICCAI 2016, Part II. LNCS, vol. 9901, pp. 424–432. Springer, Cham (2016). https://doi.org/10.1007/978-3-319-46723-8_49
3. Fox, C.R., Rottenstreich, Y.: Partition priming in judgment under uncertainty. Psychol. Sci. **14**(3), 195–200 (2003)
4. Gal, Y., Ghahramani, Z.: Dropout as a Bayesian approximation: representing model uncertainty in deep learning. In: Proceedings of the 33rd International Conference on Machine Learning, ICML 2016 (2016)
5. Gal, Y., Islam, R., Ghahramani, Z.: Deep Bayesian active learning with image data. In: Proceedings of the 34th International Conference on Machine Learning, ICML 2017, Sydney, NSW, Australia, 6–11 August 2017, pp. 1183–1192 (2017)
6. Huang, L., Pashler, H.: Symmetry detection and visual attention: a "binary-map" hypothesis. Vis. Res. **42**(11), 1421–1430 (2002)
7. Jungo, A., et al.: On the effect of inter-observer variability for a reliable estimation of uncertainty of medical image segmentation. In: Frangi, A.F., Schnabel, J.A., Davatzikos, C., Alberola-López, C., Fichtinger, G. (eds.) MICCAI 2018, Part I. LNCS, vol. 11070, pp. 682–690. Springer, Cham (2018). https://doi.org/10.1007/978-3-030-00928-1_77
8. Kamnitsas, K., et al.: Efficient multi-scale 3D CNN with fully connected CRF for accurate brain lesion segmentation. Med. Image Anal. **36**, 61–78 (2017)
9. Kendall, A., Badrinarayanan, V., Cipolla, R.: Bayesian SegNet: model uncertainty in deep convolutional encoder-decoder architectures for scene understanding. In: British Machine Vision Conference 2017, BMVC 2017, London, UK, 4–7 September 2017 (2017)
10. Kohl, S., et al.: A probabilistic U-Net for segmentation of ambiguous images. In: Advances in Neural Information Processing Systems 31: Annual Conference on Neural Information Processing Systems 2018, NeurIPS 2018, Montréal, Canada, 3–8 December 2018, pp. 6965–6975 (2018)
11. Mobiny, A., Nguyen, H.V., Moulik, S., Garg, N., Wu, C.C.: DropConnect Is Effective in Modeling Uncertainty of Bayesian Deep Networks. arXiv preprint arXiv:1906.04569 (2019)
12. Nair, T., Precup, D., Arnold, D.L., Arbel, T.: Exploring uncertainty measures in deep networks for multiple sclerosis lesion detection and segmentation. In: Frangi, A.F., Schnabel, J.A., Davatzikos, C., Alberola-López, C., Fichtinger, G. (eds.) MICCAI 2018, Part I. LNCS, vol. 11070, pp. 655–663. Springer, Cham (2018). https://doi.org/10.1007/978-3-030-00928-1_74

13. Ronneberger, O., Fischer, P., Brox, T.: U-Net: convolutional networks for biomedical image segmentation. In: Navab, N., Hornegger, J., Wells, W.M., Frangi, A.F. (eds.) MICCAI 2015. LNCS, vol. 9351, pp. 234–241. Springer, Cham (2015). https://doi.org/10.1007/978-3-319-24574-4_28

14. Roy, A.G., Conjeti, S., Navab, N., Wachinger, C.: Inherent brain segmentation quality control from fully ConvNet Monte Carlo sampling. In: Frangi, A.F., Schnabel, J.A., Davatzikos, C., Alberola-López, C., Fichtinger, G. (eds.) MICCAI 2018, Part I. LNCS, vol. 11070, pp. 664–672. Springer, Cham (2018). https://doi.org/10.1007/978-3-030-00928-1_75

15. Sakaridis, C., Dai, D., Van Gool, L.: Semantic nighttime image segmentation with synthetic stylized data, gradual adaptation and uncertainty-aware evaluation. arXiv preprint arXiv:1901.05946 (2019)

16. Smith, L., Gal, Y.: Understanding measures of uncertainty for adversarial example detection. In: Proceedings of the Thirty-Fourth Conference on Uncertainty in Artificial Intelligence, UAI 2018, Monterey, California, USA, 6–10 August 2018, pp. 560–569 (2018)

17. Sohn, K., Lee, H., Yan, X.: Learning structured output representation using deep conditional generative models. In: Advances in Neural Information Processing Systems, pp. 3483–3491 (2015)

18. Wang, S., et al.: Central focused convolutional neural networks: developing a data-driven model for lung nodule segmentation. Med. Image Anal. **40**, 172–183 (2017)

DeepIGeoS-V2: Deep Interactive Segmentation of Multiple Organs from Head and Neck Images with Lightweight CNNs

Wenhui Lei[1], Huan Wang[1], Ran Gu[1], Shichuan Zhang[2], Shaoting Zhang[1], and Guotai Wang[1(✉)]

[1] School of Mechanical and Electrical Engineering,
University of Electronic Science and Technology of China, Chengdu, China
guotai.wang@uestc.edu.cn
[2] Department of Radiation Oncology, Sichuan Cancer Hospital and Institute,
University of Electronic Science and Technology of China, Chengdu, China

Abstract. Accurate segmentation of organs-at-risks (OARs) from Computed Tomography (CT) image is a key step for efficient planning of radiation therapy for nasopharyngeal carcinoma (NPC) treatment. Convolutional Neural Networks (CNN) have recently become the state-of-the-art automated OARs image segmentation method. However, due to the low contrast of head and neck organism tissues in CT, the fully automatic segmentation may still need to be refined to become accurate and robust enough for clinical use. We propose a deep learning-based multi-organ interactive segmentation method to improve the results obtained by an automatic CNN and to reduce user interactions during refinement for higher accuracy. We use one CNN to obtain an initial automatic segmentation, on which user interactions are added to indicate mis-segmentation. Another CNN takes as input the user interactions with the initial segmentation and gives a refined result. We propose a dimension separate lightweight network that gives a faster and better dense predictions. In addition, we propose a mis-segmentation-based weighting strategy combined with loss functions to achieve more accurate segmentation. We validated the proposed framework in the context of 3D head and neck organism segmentation from CT images. Experimental results show our method achieves a large improvement from automatic CNNs, and obtains higher accuracy with fewer user interventions and less time compared with traditional interactive segmentation method.

1 Introduction

Nasopharyngeal carcinoma (NPC) is a malignant tumor prevalent globally [5]. Radiotherapy is one of the main treatments for NPC. Segmentation of organs-at-risks (OARs) from Computed Tomography (CT) images is a key step for efficient planning of radiotherapy, which is usually undertaken by radiation

© Springer Nature Switzerland AG 2019
L. Zhou et al. (Eds.): LABELS 2019/HAL-MICCAI 2019/CuRIOUS 2019, LNCS 11851, pp. 61–69, 2019.
https://doi.org/10.1007/978-3-030-33642-4_7

therapists with laborious manual delineation. Recently, deep learning with convolutional neural networks (CNNs) has achieved state-of-the-art performance for automated OARs image segmentation [3,4]. However, they can rarely achieve sufficiently accurate and robust results to be useful for accurate planning of radiotherapy due to CT images' low contrast of soft tissues, variations among patients, and the tiny sizes of organs like optic nerve and optic chaism. Alternatively, interactive segmentation methods can integrate the human experts' knowledge with machine intelligence to improve segmentation accuracy and efficiency [11].

Traditional interactive segmentation methods such as Graph Cut [1] and ITK-SNAP [10] are usually applicable for segmentation of well-circumscribed objects. However, since they are low-level feature-based, these methods require a large number of user interactions to obtain good results when dealing with a stack of medical images, which will increase the burden on the user. Motivated by these observations, we investigate combining CNNs with user interactions for multi-organ segmentation from medical images to achieve higher segmentation accuracy and robustness with fewer user interactions and less user time. However, there have been very few studies on using CNNs for interactive segmentation [7,8] and they are all proposed for a single object segmentation rather than multiple organs. DeepIGeoS [8], for example, combines user interactions with CNNs via geodesic distance transforms to obtain higher accuracy for medical image segmentation but it was not designed for multi-organ segmentation.

This paper aims to integrate user interactions into CNN frameworks for efficient segmentation of multiple OARs (brain stem, parotid gland, optic nerve and optic chaism) from 3D CT images. We aim to make the interactive framework more efficient with a minimal number of user interactions by using CNNs. In addition, to achieve fast response to user interactions, the CNN frameworks should be small and fast enough for clinical applications with high accuracy and efficiency.

The contributions of this work are three-fold. (1) We propose a deep CNN-based interactive framework for multiple OARs segmentation from 3D CT images. Compared with previous works [7,8] that use CNNs for binary interactive segmentation, our method can obtain segmentation of multiple organs simultaneously; (2) For efficient interactive segmentation, we propose a lightweight CNN structure based on 3D-Unet [2], which could achieve accurate segmentation in real-time; (3) We present a new mis-segmentation-based weighting strategy combined with loss functions to get more room for network improvement and focus more on the mis-segmented regions. We show that this new weighting strategy can lead to improved segmentation accuracy. Experimental results show that our proposed method outperforms existing interactive tools for segmentation of multiple organs at risk from CT images.

2   Methodology

DeepIGeoS [8] was an efficient framework for interactive segmentation of binary objects. However, it cannot deal with multiple organs and uses a dense network

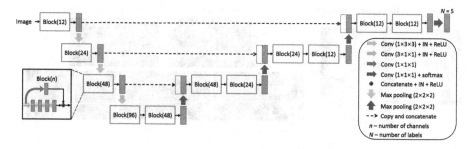

Fig. 1. Proposed lightweight network architecture optimized for 3D segmentation.

structure that may limit its response speed. To address these problems, we extend DeepIGeoS [8] by dealing with multi-organ segmentation with a lightweight network (L-Net) that improves response speed and a mis-segmentation-aware loss function. The framework consists of two main stages. First, an initial segmentation proposal network (L-Net1) takes as input a raw image with one channel and gives an initial segmentation of N classes ($N = 5$ in our case). Then the interactions (clicks or scribbles) are provided by the users to indicate mis-segmented regions of one or more classes. Second, a refine network (L-Net2) takes as input the original image, the initial segmentation and user interactions to provide a refined segmentation. Based on the initial automatic segmentation obtained by L-Net1, the user could give clicks/scribbles to refine the result more than one time through L-Net2.

Proposed Lightweight Network Architecture. Considering that user interactions are required for multiple organs and the segmentation may be refined for multiple times, real-time response to user interactions is highly required. Therefore we explore lightweight CNNs that can obtain accurate segmentation with high speed. Our network is a variant of 3D-Unet [2], and composed of 11 convolutional blocks. Our CT images have an in-plane resolution of around 1.0 mm × 1.0 mm with slice-spacing 3.0 mm. We separate 3D convolutions into $3 \times 3 \times 1$ intra-slice convolutions and $1 \times 1 \times 3$ inter-slice convolutions. Each block comprises 3/1 cascading $1 \times 3 \times 3 / 3 \times 1 \times 1$ convolutional layers of n channels associated with instance normalization (IN) [6] and rectified linear units (ReLU). A skip connection with a $1 \times 1 \times 1$ convolutional layer is used in each block for better convergence. The number of channels (n) is doubled after each max pooling and is halved after each upsampling. We concatenate feature maps from the encoding path with the corresponding feature maps in the decoding path for better convergence. A final layer of $1 \times 1 \times 1$ convolution with the softmax function provides the segmentation probabilities, as shown in Fig. 1. L-Net1 and L-Net2 share the same structure except the difference in the number of input channels.

Encoding User Interactions Through Distance Transformation. In our method, the users provide scribbles to refine the initial automatic segmentation

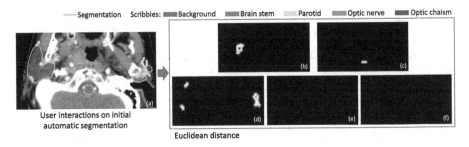

Fig. 2. The Euclidean distance transforms of user interactions. (a) The user provides clicks/scribbles to correct background(red) and organisms(others) on the initial automatic segmentation.(b), (c), (d), (e) and (f) are Euclidean distance map for the background and brain stem, parotid, optic nerve, optic chaism respectively. (Color figure online)

obtained by L-Net1. A scribble labels a set of pixels as background or one of the 4 organisms, with 5 classes totally. Interactions with the same label are converted into a distance map, 5 maps totally. In [8], the geodesic distance was used due to it helps to better differentiate neighboring pixels with different appearances, and improve label consistency in homogeneous regions. However, in our case, some of the head-neck organisms have a low contrast to the neighbouring tissues, e.g. brain stem. Their geodesic distance maps could help little to tell the difference between a target organ and neighboring tissues. For simplicity, we propose to encode user interactions via Euclidean distance transforms for CNN-based segmentation.

Suppose S_c represents the set of pixels labeled by scribbles for class $c \in [0, 4]$, respectively. Let $\boldsymbol{x}$ be a pixel position in an image $\mathbf{I}$, then the unsigned Euclidean distance from $\boldsymbol{x}$ to the scribble set S_c is:

$$D_{euc}(\boldsymbol{x}, \boldsymbol{y}, \mathbf{I}) = \min(\sqrt{\sum_{i}^{n} d_i^2 (\boldsymbol{x}_i - \boldsymbol{y}_i)^2}, T_c) \tag{1}$$

$$E(\boldsymbol{x}, S_c, \mathbf{I}) = 1 - \min_{\boldsymbol{y} \in S_c} D_{euc}(\boldsymbol{x}, \boldsymbol{y}, \mathbf{I})/T_c \tag{2}$$

where n is the dimension of image $\mathbf{I}$. d_i is the pixel spacing along the i-th dimension. T_c represents the upper bound of Euclidean distance of class c, and we set $[T_0, T_1, T_3, T_3, T_4] = [4, 4, 4, 2, 2]$ pixels for background, brain stem, parotid, optic nerve and optic chaism. As shown in Eq. 2, we use a normalized Euclidean distance E in the range of [0, 1], and a higher value of E represents a higher possibility of pixel $\boldsymbol{x}$ belonging to class c.

Figure 2 shows an example of Euclidean distance transforms of user interactions. The Euclidean distance maps of user interactions and the initial automatic segmentation have the same size as $\mathbf{I}$. They are concatenated with the raw channels of $\mathbf{I}$ and the automatic segmentation, which is a single-channel image where the pixel value representing the class predicted by L-Net1. Therefore the refinement network L-Net2 accepts a concatenated image with 7 channels as the input.

Attention to Mis-Segmentation. Mis-segmentation information is important for guiding the network where to pay more attention to. It's meaningful to weight the mis-segmented regions in loss functions, forcing the network to focus on the hard regions. More formally, we propose to multiply the prediction result by a weight function, with tunable *attentional* parameter $\alpha > 0$. We define the weight function as:

$$w_c(\boldsymbol{x}) = e^{\frac{p_c(\boldsymbol{x}) - g_c(\boldsymbol{x})}{\alpha}} \qquad (3)$$

and the weighted prediction is represented as:

$$p_c^w(\boldsymbol{x}) = p_c(\boldsymbol{x})w_c(\boldsymbol{x}) \qquad (4)$$

where $\boldsymbol{x}$ is the pixel position and c is the label. $p_c(\boldsymbol{x})$ is the softmax probability representing the probability of pixel $\boldsymbol{x}$ belonging to class c. $g_c(\boldsymbol{x}) \in 0, 1$ is the ground truth probability for pixel $\boldsymbol{x}$ being class c. The $p_c^w(\boldsymbol{x})$ is the weighted prediction, and a higher value of $p_c^w(\boldsymbol{x})$ represents a higher possibility of pixel $\boldsymbol{x}$ belonging to class c. It is visualized for several values of $\alpha \in [0, 2]$ in Fig. 3. We notice the $p_c^w(\boldsymbol{x})$ is lower than $p_c(\boldsymbol{x})$ for $g_c(\boldsymbol{x}) = 1$ and higher for $g_c(\boldsymbol{x}) = 0$, meaning the weighted prediction is further away from the ground truth. As a result, the weighted mis-segmented region will have a larger impact on backpropagation as they have larger gradient values than correctly predicted voxels. Generally, it can get more room for improvement and have the network focus more on the mis-segmented regions. It should be noticed that this weighted function needs to be combined with a loss function in training progress and we combine it with exponential logarithmic loss [9] in our case, named $ATM - L_{Exp}$.

Training Strategy. For pre-processing, all images were normalized by the mean value and standard variation. Random cropping was used for data augmentation. We implemented L-Net1 and L-Net2 using our proposed lightweight structure in PyTorch, and trained them on two NVIDIA 1080ti GPUs. Batch size was set to be 16. The optimizer Adam was used with the learning rate as 10^{-3}, weight decay 10^{-8}, and 200 epochs. The learning rate was decayed by 0.9 every 10 epochs for L-Net1 and 0.7 for L-Net2.

After the training of L-Net1, we automatically simulated user interactions to train L-Net2. The automatic segmentation of training images was compared with the ground truth to find mis-segmented regions. Then the user interactions on each under-segmented region of class c were simulated by randomly sampling a pixels in that region. Note that an over-segmentation of one certain class can be regarded as an under-segmentation of another class. Suppose the size of one connected under-segmented region for class c was N_m, we set a for that region to 0 if $N_m < 30$ and $N_m/100$ otherwise based on experience. These sampled pixels for class c were converted to the distance map for class c via Euclidean distance transforms.

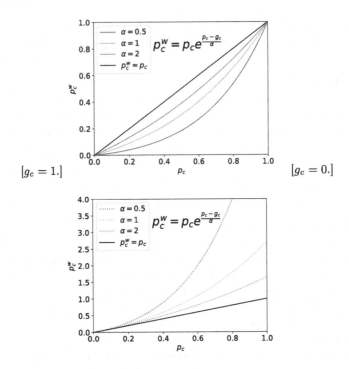

Fig. 3. Weighted prediction with different α and g_c.

3   Experiments

Experimental Data and Evaluation Method. We collected HaN CT images from 73 patients with nasopharyngeal carcinoma before radiotherapy treatment with slice dimension 512×512, voxel spacing $0.9766\,\text{mm} \times 0.9766\,\text{mm}$, slice thickness $3\,\text{mm}$. They were manually segmented by a experienced Radiologist. Each segmentation contained brain stem, parotid, optic nerve and optic chaism, thus 5 labels with background included. We removed the chest region from CT images and cropped a box of size 256×256 containing the cerebrum to focus on head and neck anatomies. The dataset was randomly split to 70% for training, 10% for validation and 20% for test. We used Dice coefficient (DSC) and Average Symmetric Surface Distance (ASSD) for quantitative evalution.

Automatic Segmentation by L-Net1. We compare our proposed lightweight network with 3D-Unet for automatic segmentation in the first stage, and also compare the performance of different loss functions: Dice loss, exponential logarithmic loss (L_{Exp}) [9], and our proposed attention to mis-segmentation(ATM) with L_{Exp}, which is refered to as $ATM - L_{Exp}$. The results are shown in Table 1. It can be observed that L-Net1 trained with $ATM - L_{Exp}$ with $\alpha = 0.5$ achieves better results than the other loss functions. We also used the same types of loss functions to train the 3D-Unet [2], whose parameter number is three times larger than that of L-Net1, and its performance is only slightly better than that of L-Net1. It shows L-Net1 could obtain accurate segmentation with a lightweight structure. For each patient in the experiment, it takes less than 0.26 s to get the result averagely, with a 3-time speedup compared with 3D-Unet. However, there are still some obvious mis-segmented regions by L-Net1 as shown in Fig. 4. Therefore we use L-Net2 to refine the segmentation interactively in the following.

Table 1. Quantitative comparison of different network structures and loss functions for automatic segmentation in stage 1 of our method, evaluated with Dice coefficients and ASSD (format: mean ± std%, mean ± std pixels).

Net	Loss Function	Brain Stem	Parotid	Optic Nerve	Optic Chaism
L-Net1	Dice loss	78.71±3.72,2.61±1.71	79.63±4.93,3.28±1.62	52.26±12.25,1.72±0.75	36.12±12.34,2.27±0.58
	L_{Exp}	75.50±4.70,2.91±0.67	79.84±3.18,1.97±0.40	54.94±7.37,1.97±1.47	35.24±14.14,2.21±0.74
	$ATM(\alpha = 0.5) - L_{Exp}$	**85.56±2.55**,1.49±0.37	**81.54±4.88,1.76±0.66**	62.75±5.92,**1.11±0.33**	37.74±12.35,**2.04±0.75**
	$ATM(\alpha = 1) - L_{Exp}$	84.32±2.78,1.70±0.45	81.22±4.08,1.80±0.51	63.18±7.40,1.46±1.59	37.52±11.79,2.07±0.74
	$ATM(\alpha = 2) - L_{Exp}$	78.73±3.52,2.57±0.54	80.06±4.42,2.22±0.99	**63.42±8.66**,1.54±1.63	**37.78±12.96**,2.07±0.77
3D-Unet	Dice loss	81.54±3.37,1.80±1.19	79.03±5.03,1.97±0.80	62.47±5.35,0.94±0.57	36.88±10.33,1.44±0.44
	L_{Exp}	78.07±6.08,2.42±1.34	76.93±3.67,2.22±0.81	60.63±9.26,1.24±0.67	37.79±16.08,1.58±0.98
	$ATM(\alpha = 0.5) - L_{Exp}$	83.18±2.68,1.09±0.17	82.75±2.86,1.23±0.32	64.76±7.94,0.83±0.70	40.92±13.60,1.25±0.54
	$ATM(\alpha = 1) - L_{Exp}$	79.97±4.75,1.44±0.49	74.77±4.04,3.48±1.39	62.37±6.55,0.80±0.34	37.01±14.72,1.51±0.64
	$ATM(\alpha = 2) - L_{Exp}$	80.20±4.88,1.91±1.07	76.52±3.31,1.96±0.55	61.35±6.79,0.95±0.40	36.86±15.63,1.52±0.77

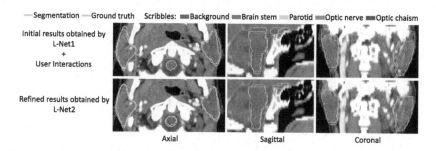

Fig. 4. Visual comparison of automatic and refined segmentation. The first row shows the initial automatic segmentation obtained by L-Net1 and user interactions added for refinement. The second row shows refined results by L-Net2.

Refined Segmentation by L-Net2. Figure 4 shows examples of auto and refined segmentation based on L-Net1 and L-Net2 trained with $ATM - L_{Exp}$ with $\alpha = 0.5$. The first row in Fig. 4 shows initial segmentation results obtained by L-Net1. The user provides clicks/scribbles to indicate the background or the organisms. The second row in Fig. 4 shows the results refined by L-Net2. We measured the segmentation accuracy after iterations of user refinement (giving user interactions to mark the main mis-segmented regions and applying refinement). The results are presented in Table 2, showing the L-Net2 leads to more accurate segmentation with user interactions.

Comparison with ITK-SNAP. Currently traditional multi-class interactive segmentation methods mainly based on low level features may not be appropriate to segmentation of head and neck organism tissues in CT due to their low contrast and we choose one of the most famous method to show it. We compared our proposed DeepIGeoS-V2 with the widely used interactive segmentation tool ITK-SNAP [10]. A user was asked to use these two tools to segment all the testing images respectively. For ITK-SNAP, the OARs were segmented one after another as it only supports binary segmentation. We evaluate the effectiveness of these methods in terms of user time and final accuracy that are the two most straightforward metrics for interactive methods [8]. The results are demonstrated in Fig. 5, which shows that DeepIGeoS-V2 achieve higher accuracy with about half of user time compared with ITK-SNAP.

Table 2. The results of refined segmentation, evaluated with Dice coefficients and ASSD (format: mean $\pm$ std%, mean $\pm$ std pixels). L-Net1 and L-Net2 in two stages were trained with $ATM(\alpha = 0.5) - L_{Exp}$.

Method	Brain Stem	Parotid	Optic Nerve	Optic Chaism
Before refinement	85.56±2.55,1.49±0.37	81.54±4.88,1.76±0.66	62.75±5.92,1.11±0.33	37.74±12.35,2.04±0.75
After refinement	**86.60±2.18,1.17±0.23**	**85.71±3.50,1.58±0.522**	**66.40±5.95,0.95±0.27**	**52.59±8.11,1.29±0.39**

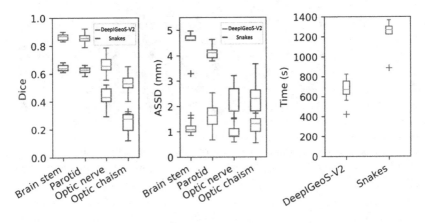

Fig. 5. Accuracy and user time comparison between our proposed DeepIGeoS-V2 and ITK-SNAP for interactive segmentation of OARs from HaN CT images.

4   Conclusions

In this work, we proposed a novel 3D interactive framework for 3D segmentation of multiple organs from head and neck CT images. We extend the two-stage pipeline of DeepIGeoS [8] to deal with multiple organs. We also proposed a lightweight CNN and a mis-segmentation-based weighting strategy combined with loss functions to focus on the mis-segment regions and to get more room for performance improvement. Segmentation results of the head and neck organisms CT images show that our proposed method achieves better results than automatic CNNs. It requires far less user time and achieves higher accuracy for 3D head and neck organisms segmentation compared with traditional interactive methods. This work has the potential to facilitate more efficient and accurate segmentation of OARs from CT images for radiotherapy planning of NPC. In the future, it is of interest to apply our framework to some other multi-organ segmentation tasks, such as interactive segmentation of multiple abdominal organs.

References

1. Boykov, Y.Y., Jolly, M.P.: Interactive graph cuts for optimal boundary & region segmentation of objects in ND images. In: ICCV, pp. 105–112 (2001)
2. Çiçek, Ö., Abdulkadir, A., Lienkamp, S.S., Brox, T., Ronneberger, O.: 3D U-Net: learning dense volumetric segmentation from sparse annotation. In: Ourselin, S., Joskowicz, L., Sabuncu, M.R., Unal, G., Wells, W. (eds.) MICCAI 2016. LNCS, vol. 9901, pp. 424–432. Springer, Cham (2016). https://doi.org/10.1007/978-3-319-46723-8_49
3. Ibragimov, B., Xing, L.: Segmentation of organs-at-risks in head and neck CT images using convolutional neural networks. Med. Phys. **44**(2), 547–557 (2017)
4. Raudaschl, P.F., et al.: Evaluation of segmentation methods on head and neck CT: auto-segmentation challenge 2015. Med. Phys. **44**(5), 2020–2036 (2017)
5. Torre, L.A., Bray, F., Siegel, R.L., Ferlay, J., Lortet-Tieulent, J., Jemal, A.: Global cancer statistics, 2012. CA Cancer J. Clin. **65**(2), 87–108 (2015)
6. Ulyanov, D., Vedaldi, A., Lempitsky, V.: Instance normalization: the missing ingredient for fast stylization. arXiv preprint arXiv:1607.08022 (2016)
7. Wang, G., et al.: Interactive medical image segmentation using deep learning with image-specific fine tuning. IEEE TMI **37**(7), 1562–1573 (2018)
8. Wang, G., et al.: DeepiGeoS: a deep interactive geodesic framework for medical image segmentation. In: IEEE TPAMI (2018)
9. Wong, K.C., Moradi, M., Tang, H., Syeda-Mahmood, T.: 3D segmentation with exponential logarithmic loss for highly unbalanced object sizes. In: MICCAI, pp. 612–619 (2018)
10. Yushkevich, P.A., et al.: User-guided 3D active contour segmentation of anatomical structures: significantly improved efficiency and reliability. Neuroimage **31**(3), 1116–1128 (2006)
11. Zhao, F., Xie, X.: An overview of interactive medical image segmentation. Ann. BMVA **2013**(7), 1–22 (2013)

The Role of Publicly Available Data in MICCAI Papers from 2014 to 2018

Nicholas Heller[✉], Jack Rickman, Christopher Weight, and Nikolaos Papanikolopoulos

University of Minnesota – Twin Cities, Minneapolis, USA
{helle246,rickm014,cjweight,papan001}@umn.edu

Abstract. Widely-used public benchmarks are of huge importance to computer vision and machine learning research, especially with the computational resources required to reproduce state of the art results quickly becoming untenable. In medical image computing, the wide variety of image modalities and problem formulations yields a huge task-space for benchmarks to cover, and thus the widespread adoption of standard benchmarks has been slow, and barriers to releasing medical data exacerbate this issue. In this paper, we examine the role that publicly available data has played in MICCAI papers from the past five years. We find that more than half of these papers are based on private data alone, although this proportion seems to be decreasing over time. Additionally, we observed that after controlling for open access publication and the release of code, papers based on public data were cited over 60% more per year than their private-data counterparts. Further, we found that more than 20% of papers using public data did not provide a citation to the dataset or associated manuscript, highlighting the "second-rate" status that data contributions often take compared to theoretical ones. We conclude by making recommendations for MICCAI policies which could help to better incentivise data sharing and move the field toward more efficient and reproducible science.

1 Introduction

With the proliferation of Deep Learning (DL) methods in medical image computing, a large proportion of papers presented at the International Conference on Medical Image Computing and Computer Assisted Interventions (MICCAI) are now based on large-scale medical imaging datasets which are often expensive and time-consuming to collect. In the broader computer vision community, there is a trend toward the use of standardized benchmarks such as CIFAR [11], ImageNet [4], and MSCOCO [12] which allows for researchers to objectively compare their methods to the state of the art without having to repeat the experiments of others–a time-consuming and expensive endeavor on its own. At MICCAI, this has seen only modest adoption, possibly due to the exceptional diversity of imaging modalities and target variables [8], and the corresponding dearth of publicly available benchmarks.

© Springer Nature Switzerland AG 2019
L. Zhou et al. (Eds.): LABELS 2019/HAL-MICCAI 2019/CuRIOUS 2019, LNCS 11851, pp. 70–77, 2019.
https://doi.org/10.1007/978-3-030-33642-4_8

The practice of publicly releasing research data, especially in a recognized archive accompanied by a detailed data descriptor, is a promising avenue for expanding the number and variety of medical imaging benchmarks. Medical data inherently has more barriers to publication (e.g. ethics standards in human subjects research, risks of leaking protected health information) than other scientific data, but these are typically not insurmountable, especially with organizations such as The Cancer Imaging Archive [2] now offering support in this area. Public datasets free machine learning researchers to focus their attention and resources on methods, and it frees their peers from having to replicate both the dataset *and* analysis when conducting reproducibility studies or building on their work.

In this paper, we explore the evolution of this practice at each MICCAI conferences of the past five years. In particular, we report the prevalence of papers based on public data vs. those based on only private data. We found that more than half of all MICCAI papers about machine learning for computer vision are based on private data alone, which is anomalously high for ML/CV literature. We also use each paper's citation count per year elapsed as a surrogate for its impact on the field and show that papers using public data are cited roughly 60% more than their private data counterparts, even when controlling for open access publication and release of code. We conclude with recommendations for how these data can inform policies to increase the impact of the MICCAI conference and the field of medical image computing as a whole.

2   Related Work

There is a large and diverse body of literature that shows the benefit of sharing research data. In a 2013 article, Piwowar and Vision [13] succinctly articulated the many benefits to publishing your data in the biomedical field:

> ... sharing data encourages multiple perspectives, helps to identify errors, discourages fraud, is useful for training new researchers, and increases efficient use of funding and patient population resources by avoiding duplicate data collection.

They then went on to provide the results of a thorough and well-controlled experiment which showed that papers that released their associated gene expression microarray data were cited nearly 10% more than their counterparts that kept the same data private.

In 2016, Drachen et al. [6] conducted a similar bibliometric analysis for three astrophysics journals between 2000 and 2014. They found that papers which linked to a dataset were cited 25% more than those that did not, and interestingly, when they restricted their analysis to only papers from 2009 to 2014, the effect size increased to 40%, which suggests that this issue is becoming more pronounced over time.

Very recently, Colavizza et al. [3] conducted a text mining and citation analysis of more than half a million papers published by PLOS and BMC that were also part of the PubMed Open Access Collection. These journals are interesting cases because they each recently enacted policies requiring authors to include a Data Availability Statement (DAS) belonging to one of three categories: (1) "data is available on request", (2) "data is contained within the article or supplementary material", and (3) "data is in a public repository and here is the link". Their results showed that papers with a category 3 DAS were cited over 25% more than those with categories 1, 2 or no DAS at all. Their work also showed that such DAS statements can very quickly be made commonplace by a change in journal policy.

These works paint a clear picture that data publication is strongly associated with receiving a higher number of citations, but what about simply *using* public data? To our knowledge, there are no published studies looking at the citation advantage to using publicly available data rather than private data.

3   Methods

3.1   Data Collection

For each of the five MICCAI events from 2014 to 2018, we randomly ordered all accepted papers, manually iterated through them and selected all papers that made use of machine learning for a computer vision task until we had accrued 100 papers from each year. We henceforth refer to such papers as "MICCAI CV/ML papers". We then manually collected the following information about each paper:

- Citation count according to Google Scholar
- Whether they used public data, and if so, which public dataset(s) they used
- How they referenced the public data they used, if applicable (e.g. citation, footnote URL, or just a name in the text)
- Whether they released the private data they used, if applicable
- Whether they released their source code
- Whether the paper is available open access (e.g. through a preprinting server, through a funding agency, or on an author's homepage)

The release of code [17] and making the paper open access [9] are known to independently associate with high citation counts, so we collected these attributes to control for potential confounding effects.

At the start of this study, we originally did not collect the manner in which data was referenced. It was only after we noticed a surprising number of non-citation references that we decided to go back and record this for our sample.

3.2   Statistical Analysis

In order to make our study of citation counts robust to the very few papers with an exceptionally high number of citations, we used Winsorization [5]. In particular, we trimmed each paper's citation rate to 50 per year. Two papers were affected by this [1,14] and the Winsorization affected neither the direction nor the significance of the results.

We are interested in estimating the mean citation advantage to using public data vs using only private data, after controlling for release of code and open access publication. Regression is not suitable in this case since the prerequisite of normal residuals fails badly. Prior works [16] have used OLS to predict the log of citations/year plus one, but this dramatically underestimates effect sizes when there is a high prevalence of low-citation papers, as there is in our case. Luckily, since we are controlling only for two binary variables, we can stratify papers into four groups without loss of precision: (1) no code release and no open access, (2) code release but not open access, (3) no code release but open access, and (4) code release and open access. Within each stratum, we compute a ratio of the mean citations per year of papers using public data to that of papers that used only private data. We then aggregate these ratios with a weighted sum according to their prevalence. In order to estimate a confidence interval for this ratio, we use the bootstrap [7].

4   Results and Discussion

4.1   More Than Half of Papers Used Only Private Data

Of the 500 papers we reviewed, 271 (54.2%) used only privately available data. It does appear, however, that even within our short study period, this practice has become less common, down from 64.0% in 2014 to 44% in 2018. See Fig. 1 for a depiction of this trend.

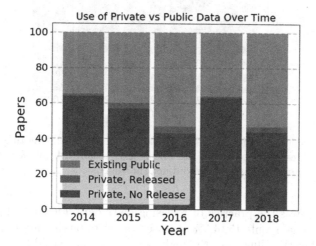

Fig. 1. The various modes of data used by MICCAI CV/ML papers from 2014 through 2018. The lightest region (top) represents papers that used at least one existing public dataset, the middle region represents papers that used their own data but publicly released it with their paper, and the darkest region (bottom) represents papers using only private data that was not released with publication.

We have no explanation for the anomalously high proportion of papers using private data at MICCAI 2017. We surmise that this is a *much* higher proportion than at other computer vision conferences such as CVPR and ICCV (although we have not collected the data to confirm this), which highlights the unique position of the medical image computing field where, in addition to the steep barriers to data release, the ratio of effort required in data collection to that in method development often seems much higher than in other applications of computer vision.

4.2   Few Papers Released Their Data or Code

Of the 500 papers we reviewed, only 36 (7.2%) released their code. While this is a discouragingly small proportion, it appears that steady progress has been made from 6% in 2014 to 9% in 2018. See Fig. 2 for a depiction of this trend. It's important to note, however, that with such small proportions each year, we are unable to reject the null hypothesis that this is just random variation over time.

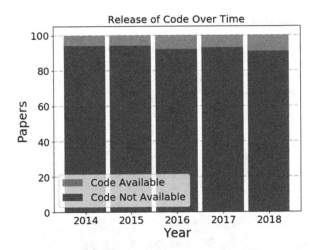

Fig. 2. The prevalence of MICCAI CV/ML papers releasing code over time. The lighter region (top) represents papers that did release their code with publications, and the darker region represents papers than did not (bottom).

Even rarer was the practice of releasing one's data. Of the 309 papers that used their own data, only 15 (4.9%) released this data by the time of publication. We believe that this illustrates the high barriers and perceived low incentives to releasing medical imaging data.

4.3   Papers Using Public Data Were Cited More Than 60% More

Among the four strata corresponding to open access or not and code release or not, the use of a public dataset (i.e. existing public or released with publication) was associated with 60.8% more citations per year than their private-data-only counterparts (95% CI: 28.1%–110.2%). Such a large effect is highly surprising, considering that prior studies in other fields [3, 6, 13] have found that *releasing* one's data is associated with only a 10%–30% increase in citations, where our study found a much larger effect from simply *using* public data. In our view, this illustrates the outsized importance of data in machine learning research, and suggests that the medical image computing field is highly catalyzed by the public release of imaging data. Of important note, however, is that due to limitations with our experimental design, we were unable to control for author reputation, which is also known to associate with citations [15]. We leave this to future work, and we thus stop short of making a causal claim about the association between public data use and citation count. However, we still believe that this association is of interest and warrants future study, especially due to its size.

4.4 More Than Quarter of Data References Were Not Citations

It follows from Sects. 4.1–4.3 that the medical image computing community stands to benefit considerably from widespread data release practices. Unfortunately, as seen in Sect. 4.2, this has yet to take hold. One potential contributing factor to this is that many seem to believe that data is not a standalone scientific contribution. In our sample, of the 218 papers that used at least one existing public dataset, 47 (21.6%) referenced a dataset in some way other than a citation (e.g. with a footnote or simply a mention of its name). This is not always the fault of the MICCAI authors, since in 11 instances (5.0%), the datasets did not have an indexed entity available to cite! If the medical image computing community is to effectively capitalize on the many benefits of public data, the following two things must happen:

1. Dataset creators must do better at archiving research data in such a way that they *can* receive due academic credit. Publicly funded archives such as The Cancer Imaging Archive [2] and PhysioNet [10] are ideal for indexing and serving this data. Additionally, peer reviewed journals for data description manuscripts such as Nature's *Scientific Data* and MPDI's *Data* are a great avenue for incentivizing high-quality, detailed descriptions of data, in addition to enforcing that the data be added to a suitable archive. These are all in line with the wider initiative to make more research data FAIR (Findable, Accessible, Interoperable, and Re-usable) [18].
2. Data users must do better to properly reference datasets and/or data description manuscripts such that the creators *do* receive academic credit. Concretely, naming a benchmark should be accompanied by a formal reference, and footnotes should be accompanied by citations whenever possible. To ensure this, reviewers and editors must be vigilant for–and stringent about– inadequate data references.

We return now to Colavizza et al. and their study of Data Availability Statements. In PLOS One, where most of the articles in their study came from, a policy was enacted in 2014 to require a DAS from each accepted paper, even if it was simply category 1 ("data is available on request"). In the course of two years, PLOS One articles went from virtually no articles with a DAS (2013) to more than half of articles (2015) having a DAS of category 2 or 3, (those are "data within the article" and "data in a repository" respectively). We posit that the MICCAI Proceedings would benefit from a similar policy, possibly not as dramatically nor as quickly due to the unique barriers we face, but it is likely to accelerate our progress toward more efficient and reproducible science.

5   Conclusion

In our study of a sample of MICCAI papers that used machine learning for computer vision from 2014 through 2018, we found that a large proportion of papers (54.2%) made use of privately available data alone. In addition, we showed that even after controlling for release of code and open access publishing, the use of publicly available data was associated with receiving more than 60% more citations per year than the use of private data alone. We noted also that a surprising proportion (21.6%) of papers using public data referenced that data in some way other than a citation, for instance a footnote with a URL, or just a name. We noticed that this was due in part to the fact that in several instances (5.0%), no entity for the dataset in question was available to cite.

Based on these findings, we recommend that measures be taken to encourage the sharing of data and to ensure that the adequate credit is awarded to those who release data that is then reused. In particular, we recommend that reviewers be instructed to inspect data references and call out instances where the reference is inadequate. We also recommend that MICCAI enact a policy requiring authors to make a short statement about the availability of their data (DAS), even if that statement is "our data cannot be made available due to [legitimate reason]".

The code and data for this study has been made available at https://github.com/neheller/labels19.

Acknowledgements. Research reported in this publication was supported by the National Cancer Institute of the National Institutes of Health under Award Number R01CA225435. The content is solely the responsibility of the authors and does not necessarily represent the official views of the National Institutes of Health.

References

1. Çiçek, Ö., Abdulkadir, A., Lienkamp, S.S., Brox, T., Ronneberger, O.: 3D U-net: learning dense volumetric segmentation from sparse annotation. In: Ourselin, S., Joskowicz, L., Sabuncu, M.R., Unal, G., Wells, W. (eds.) MICCAI 2016. LNCS, vol. 9901, pp. 424–432. Springer, Cham (2016). https://doi.org/10.1007/978-3-319-46723-8_49
2. Clark, K., et al.: The cancer imaging archive (tcia): maintaining and operating a public information repository. J. Digit. Imaging **26**(6), 1045–1057 (2013)

3. Colavizza, G., Hrynaszkiewicz, I., Staden, I., Whitaker, K., McGillivray, B.: The citation advantage of linking publications to research data. arXiv preprint arXiv:1907.02565 (2019)
4. Deng, J., Dong, W., Socher, R., Li, L.J., Li, K., Fei-Fei, L.: Imagenet: a large-scale hierarchical image database. In: 2009 IEEE Conference on Computer Vision and Pattern Recognition, pp. 248–255. IEEE (2009)
5. Dixon, W.J., Yuen, K.K.: Trimming and winsorization: a review. Statistische Hefte 15(2–3), 157–170 (1974)
6. Drachen, T., Ellegaard, O., Larsen, A., Dorch, S.: Sharing data increases citations. Liber Q. 26(2) (2016)
7. Efron, B., Tibshirani, R.J.: An Introduction to the Bootstrap. CRC Press, Boca Raton (1994)
8. Erickson, B.J., Korfiatis, P., Akkus, Z., Kline, T.L.: Machine learning for medical imaging. Radiographics 37(2), 505–515 (2017)
9. Eysenbach, G.: Citation advantage of open access articles. PLoS Biol. 4(5), e157 (2006)
10. Goldberger, A.L., Amaral, L.A., Glass, L., Hausdorff, J.M., Ivanov, P.C., Mark, R.G., Mietus, J.E., Moody, G.B., Peng, C.K., Stanley, H.E.: Physiobank, physiotoolkit, and physionet: components of a new research resource for complex physiologic signals. Circulation 101(23), e215–e220 (2000)
11. Krizhevsky, A., Hinton, G., et al.: Learning multiple layers of features from tiny images. Technical report, Citeseer (2009)
12. Lin, T.-Y., et al.: Microsoft COCO: common objects in context. In: Fleet, D., Pajdla, T., Schiele, B., Tuytelaars, T. (eds.) ECCV 2014. LNCS, vol. 8693, pp. 740–755. Springer, Cham (2014). https://doi.org/10.1007/978-3-319-10602-1_48
13. Piwowar, H.A., Vision, T.J.: Data reuse and the open data citation advantage. PeerJ 1, e175 (2013)
14. Roth, H.R., et al.: DeepOrgan: multi-level deep convolutional networks for automated pancreas segmentation. In: Navab, N., Hornegger, J., Wells, W.M., Frangi, A.F. (eds.) MICCAI 2015. LNCS, vol. 9349, pp. 556–564. Springer, Cham (2015). https://doi.org/10.1007/978-3-319-24553-9_68
15. Sekara, V., Deville, P., Ahnert, S.E., Barabási, A.L., Sinatra, R., Lehmann, S.: The chaperone effect in scientific publishing. Proc. Natl. Acad. Sci. 115(50), 12603–12607 (2018)
16. Thelwall, M., Wilson, P.: Regression for citation data: an evaluation of different methods. J. Informetrics 8(4), 963–971 (2014)
17. Vandewalle, P.: Code sharing is associated with research impact in image processing. Comput. Sci. Eng. 14(4), 42–47 (2012)
18. Wilkinson, M.D., et al.: The fair guiding principles for scientific data management and stewardship. Sci. Data 3 (2016)

First International Workshop on Hardware Aware Learning for Medical Imaging and Computer Assisted Intervention (HAL-MICCAI 2019)

Hardware Acceleration of Persistent Homology Computation

Fan Wang[1]([✉]), Chunhua Deng[2], Bo Yuan[2], and Chao Chen[1]

[1] Stony Brook University, Stony Brook, NY 11794, USA
fan.wang.1@stonybrook.edu
[2] Rutgers University, New Brunswick, NJ 08901, USA

Abstract. As a powerful tool for topological data analysis, persistent homology captures topological structures of data in a robust manner. Its pertinent information is summarized in a persistence diagram, which records topological structures, as well as their saliency. Recent years have witnessed an increased interest of persistent homology in various domains. In biomedical image analysis, persistent homology has been applied to brain images, neuron images, cardiac images and cancer pathology images. Meanwhile, the computation of persistent homology could be time-consuming due to column operations over a large matrix, called the boundary matrix. This paper seeks to accelerate persistent homology computation with a hardware implementation of the column operations of the boundary matrix. By designing a dedicated hardware to process fast matrix reduction, the proposed hardware accelerator could potentially achieve up to 20k–30k times speed-up.

Keywords: Topology data analysis · Persistent homology · Matrix operation · Hardware acceleration

1 Introduction

Topological Data Analysis studies topological structures such as connected components, handles and voids, which characterize data in a global, intuitive, and robust manner. In particular, the theory of persistent homology [8,10] captures topological properties of data through the view of a *filter function*, i.e., a scalar function such as image intensity, density function, etc. One may threshold the domain with certain threshold and inspect the *sublevel set*, namely, regions whose filter value is below the threshold. Persistent homology inspects a series of nested sublevel sets induced by different thresholds, called a filtration, and tracks the birth and death of different topological structures. The information is summarized in a persistence diagram, which is a set of points on a 2D plane whose x and y coordinates are topological structures' birth and death time respectively. See Fig. 1 for an example in which persistent homology is computed on a sample image from the MNIST dataset [13]. The sublevel sets corresponding to different function values (t_0 to t_6) are displayed with black pixels in the top row.

© Springer Nature Switzerland AG 2019
L. Zhou et al. (Eds.): LABELS 2019/HAL-MICCAI 2019/CuRIOUS 2019, LNCS 11851, pp. 81–88, 2019.
https://doi.org/10.1007/978-3-030-33642-4_9

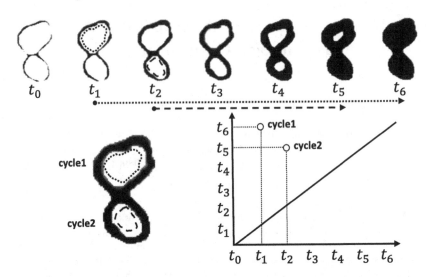

Fig. 1. Example of a persistence diagram (lower right) computed on an image (lower left) taken from the MNIST dataset. We use the inverse of the original image as input. The sublevel sets and the filtration are shown in the top row.

The upper cycle of digit 8 is created at $t1$ while the lower cycle forms at t_2. Both cycles are eventually filled in with black pixels (and thus disappear) at t_5 and t_6 respectively.

Numerous topology inspired methods have been proposed in recent years and they have been successfully applied to different problems, including molecular biology [4,12], signal analysis [18], sensor networks [11], robotics [19], shape recognition [15], graphics [7], geometric modeling [9] and many more. In biomedical image analysis, topological methods have been used but not limited to analyze global structures of sMRI and functional MRI images [1,2,14]. Topological invariant is by design robust to deformation and to noise. Without any tearing or gluing, topological structures will be preserved regardless of the deformations. A desirable property of persistence diagrams is that they are Lipschitz with respect to the underlying filter function [3].

An essential component involved in the computation of persistent homology is the reduction of a boundary matrix whose columns and rows represent elements of a discretization of a domain. Simplices of zero, one, two and three dimensions are vertices, edges, triangles and tetrahedra (Fig. 2). A boundary matrix ∂ is a binary matrix with entry $\partial(u, v) = 1$ when simplex σ_u corresponding to row u belongs to boundary of σ_v corresponding to column v. A reduction of the boundary matrix reduces it into a canonical form through column addition operations over binary field. The number of column operations required by the reduction process is usually huge, because the boundary matrices can be prohibitively large even with input images of small sizes. As an example, digit images of resolution 28×28 from MNIST have 1D boundary matrix of size 784×1512 and 2D boundary matrix of size 1512 × 729. Boundary matrix reduction has become a major bottleneck for persistent homology computation, and impedes its further applications. Therefore, it is imperative to accelerate the reduction process by dedicated hardware. Some hardware accelerators can speedup the computation process hundreds or even thousands of times compared to general purpose CPU and GPU [5,6]. By designing dedicated hardware to implement boundary matrix reduction, we can accelerate it up to 20000 times. To the best of our knowledge, this is the first paper proposing hardware accelerations for persistent homology computation.

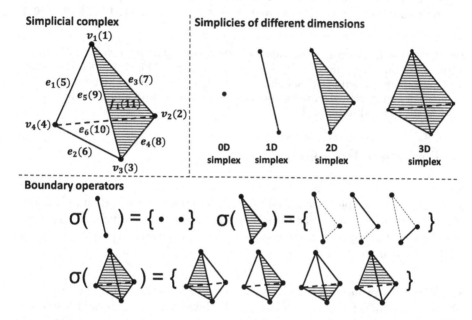

Fig. 2. Top left: a simplicial complex with filter function values marked in the parentheses beside corresponding vertices, edges, and faces; Top right: simplicies of dimension 0, 1, 2, and 3; Bottom row: examples of boundary operators on 1-, 2-, and 3-dimensional simplicies.

The remainder of the paper is organized as follows. We briefly explain the basics of the theory of persistent homology in Sect. 2. Details concerning boundary matrix and boundary matrix reduction are provided in Sect. 3. Lastly, Sect. 4 presents a hardware implementation which considerably accelerates the reduction process. Potential speedups from proposed hardware implementation are evaluated on two datasets, namely, MNIST and The Mammographic Image Analysis Society (MIAS) [20]. For illustration purpose, MIAS dataset is downsized from 1024 × 1024 to 32 × 32 with aspect ratio intact.

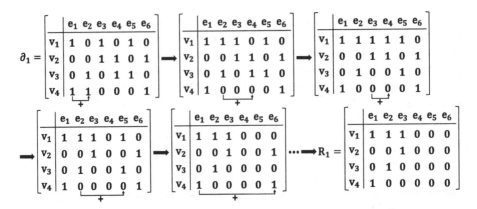

Fig. 3. ∂_1 is the 1−dimensional boundary matrix computed from the simplicial complex (with a filter function defined on it) illustrated in top left of Fig. 2. Rows and columns of ∂_1 correspond to vertices (0-simplicies) and edges (1-simplicies) respectively. First few steps of boundary matrix reduction are shown. The reduction process stops at R_1 which is the reduced result of ∂_1.

2   Persistent Homology

We review some of the basic concepts necessary to understand the idea of this paper, including simplex, simplicial complex, boundary operator, and filtration. Due to space limitations, some theories as important, such as cycle, chain group, homology group, etc., are intentionally skipped. Interested readers may refer to [10,16,17] for more details.

Simplicial Complex. A d-dimensional simplex σ is the convex hull of $d + 1$ affinely independent vertices. In case of 3D data, the 0-, 1-, 2-, and 3-simplex are vertex, edge, triangle and tetrahedron respectively (top right of Fig. 2). A simplicial complex K is a finite set of simplicies satisfying two conditions: (1) any face of a simplex in K is also in K; (2) intersection of any two simplicies in K is either empty or is a face for both simplicies.

Boundary Operator. The boundary of a d-simplex is the formal sum of the $(d − 1)$-simplicies which are faces of the d-simplex. In the second row of Fig. 2, the boundary of an edge (1-simplex) is the sum of its two endpoints (0-simplex). The edges constituting the triangle form the boundary of that triangle. And similarly, the formal sum of the four triangles is the boundary of the tetrahedron. The boundary operator is defined on individual simplicies as an operator that decomposes a d-simplex into its boundary comprising of a set of $(d−1)$-simplicies.

Filtration. Given a topology space X and a real-valued function f defined on X, we can construct a sublevel set $X_t = \{x \in X : f(x) \le t\}$ where t is a threshold controlling the "progress" of sublevel sets. As t increases from $-\infty$ to $+\infty$, a sequence of sublevel sets is produced in which the first is an empty set while the last covers the whole topology space X. This increasing sequence of sets is called a filtration induced by function f.

Algorithm 1. Boundary matrix reduction

1: **procedure** INITIALIZATION
2:     $R \leftarrow$ boundary matrix ∂
3:     $low_R() \leftarrow -1$
4: **for** $i = 1$ to n **do**
5:     **if** column i has 1 **then**
6:         $low_R(i) \leftarrow$ row index of the last 1 in column i of R
7:     **endif**
8: **endfor**
9: **for** $i = 1$ to n **do**
10:     **while** $\exists i' < i$ with $low_R(i') = low_R(i)$ **do**
11:         add column i' to column i
12:         update $low_R(i)$
13:     **endwhile**
14: **endfor**

---

3   Boundary Matrix Reduction

Computation of persistence diagram requires a filter function defined on simplicies. As can be seen from top left of Fig. 2, filtration function values are marked beside corresponding simplicies (vertices, edges, and faces). With the simplicies sorted usually in increasing order according to their function values, a boundary matrix ∂ can be computed by encoding the boundary operator in a binary matrix. An entry $\partial(u, v) = 1$ when simplex σ_u corresponding to column u is part of the boundary of simplex σ_v corresponding to column v.

Boundary matrix reduction reduces ∂ to another binary matrix R through column operations performed on ∂ from left to right. During each operation, a new column is reduced by addition with a potentially already reduced column from its left. The reduction process finishes when the rightmost column of R has index of nonzero entry as small as possible (or as high as possible in terms of matrix position) or the rightmost column is zero. To better explain the reduction, we define $low_R(i)$ to be the row index of the last 1 in column i of R or -1 in case that column i is zero. To reduce column i, we keep searching for another column j satisfying condition $low_R(i) = low_R(j), j < i$ and adding column j to column i until i is zero or no column j satisfying above condition can be found. It is important to note that these column additions use $\mathbb{Z}_2$ (i.e. mod 2) arithmetic so that $1 + 1 = 0$.

As an example, the 1−dimensional boundary matrix ∂_1 computed from the simplicial complex defined in top left of Fig. 2 is reduced with first few

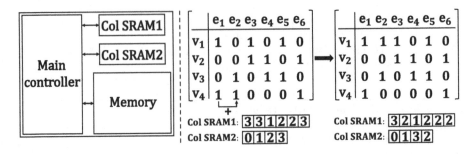

Fig. 4. Left: architecture of the proposed hardware implementation of boundary matrix reduction. Right: example Col SRAM updates of the first reduction step in Fig. 3.

steps of reduction process shown in Fig. 3. The reduced result is R_1 where $low_{R_1}(i) \neq low_{R_1}(j), i \neq j$ where column i and j specify two nonzero columns (see lower right of Fig. 3). Pseucodes for boundary matrix reduction is provided in Algorithm 1 where the boundary matrix is first scanned to initialize $low_R()$ with correct indices (the first for-loop) after which the algorithm follows what we have described previously.

4   Hardware Implementation

As described in Sect. 3, boundary matrix reduction entails a lot of column operations, which make it time-consuming to compute persistence diagram. Provided a large boundary matrix, the excessive number of cache misses caused by aforementioned column operations involved in reduction process inevitably become a major challenge in memory operations. Moreover, finding two columns i and j satisfying $low_R(i) = low_R(j)$ proves to be difficult due to the time and power consumption incurred from the perspective of both software and hardware. A novel hardware accelerator for boundary matrix reduction is proposed in this section, which can potentially achieve up to 20k–30k times speedups on MNIST and MIAS dataset.

A full description of the functionality for each hardware module illustrated in Fig. 4 is as follows:

1. Memory: the memory module stores boundary matrix. Currently, only on-chip SRAM is considered. The architecture can be easily extended to DRAM when applied to a larger dataset.
2. Col SRAM1: Col SRAM1 stores the index of the lowest 1 in each column (i.e. $low_R()$).
3. Col SRAM2: Col SRAM2 stores the number columns which share the same $low_R()$.
4. Main Controller: the main controller module is responsible for the control of the entire hardware including reading and writing of the SRAMs.

An example hardware flow of the first boundary matrix reduction step in Fig. 3 is shown in Fig. 4. Col SRAM1 indicates the index of the lowest 1 in column i (i.e. $low_R(i)$) while Col SRAM2 records the number of columns with the same $low_R()$. As the process of boundary matrix reduction progresses, the SRAMs are updated concurrently. With the information readily stored in SRAMs, the time to search for a new pair of qualifying columns can be greatly reduced.

Specifically, the Memory module is configured to have 24 SRAMs, each with depth of 1536 and width of $32-$bit in our implementation. The circuit is synthesized with 28 nm CMOS technology. The circuit is designed to have an area of $0.5\,\text{mm}^2$ and to consume 20 mW power at 1 Ghz clock frequency.

10 samples were randomly drawn from both MNIST and MIAS dataset, and we measured their software and hardware reduction time on $1-$ and $2-$ dimensional boundary matrices separately for clarity purpose. Our software implementation of boundary matrix reduction (abbreviated as SW in Table 1 for clarity) was coded in C++ and compiled on a $64-$bit Windows with Visual Studio 2015 as baseline approach. It took in filtration matrices as inputs and produced reduced boundary matrices as outputs. Additionally, software metrics reported in Table 1 were produced from a machine with an Intel Core i7-9700K 3.6 GHz CPU, and 8GB DDR4 memory. Table 1 gives averaged running time over 10 samples for both dataset, and we can observe considerable speedups from our proposed hardware accelerator especially for 1-dimensional boundary matrices.

Table 1. Comparisons of processing time between software and hardware implementations.

Dataset	Dimensions	SW runtime	HW runtime	HW/SW speedups
MNIST	2-dim	2224 ms	1.10 ms	2022x
	1-dim	2639 ms	0.13 ms	20300x
MIAS	2-dim	4087 ms	1.51 ms	2706x
	1-dim	4816 ms	0.22 ms	21891x

Acknowledgement. This work is partially supported by National Science Foundation Awards CCF-1854742, CCF-1815699, IIS-1855759 and CCF-1855760.

References

1. Chung, M.K., Bubenik, P., Kim, P.T.: Persistence diagrams of cortical surface data. In: Prince, J.L., Pham, D.L., Myers, K.J. (eds.) IPMI 2009. LNCS, vol. 5636, pp. 386–397. Springer, Heidelberg (2009). https://doi.org/10.1007/978-3-642-02498-6_32
2. Chung, M., Hanson, J., Ye, J., Davidson, R., Pollak, S.: Persistent homology in sparse regression and its application to brain morphometry. IEEE Trans. Med. Imaging **34**(9), 1928–1939 (2015). https://doi.org/10.1109/TMI.2015.2416271
3. Cohen-Steiner, D., Edelsbrunner, H., Harer, J.: Stability of persistence diagrams. Discret. Comput. Geom. **37**(1), 103–120 (2007)

4. Cohen-Steiner, D., Edelsbrunner, H., Morozov, D.: Vines and vineyards by updating persistence in linear time. In: Proceedings of the Twenty-second Annual Symposium on Computational Geometry, SCG 2006, pp. 119–126. ACM, New York (2006). https://doi.org/10.1145/1137856.1137877

5. Deng, C., Liao, S., Xie, Y., Parhi, K.K., Qian, X., Yuan, B.: PermDNN: efficient compressed DNN architecture with permuted diagonal matrices. In: 2018 51st Annual IEEE/ACM International Symposium on Microarchitecture (MICRO), pp. 189–202, October 2018. https://doi.org/10.1109/MICRO.2018.00024

6. Deng, C., Sun, F., Qian, X., Lin, J., Wang, Z., Yuan, B.: TIE: energy-efficient tensor train-based inference engine for deep neural network. In: Proceedings of the 46th International Symposium on Computer Architecture, ISCA 2019, pp. 264–278. ACM, New York (2019). https://doi.org/10.1145/3307650.3322258

7. Dey, T.K., Li, K., Sun, J., Cohen-Steiner, D.: Computing geometry-aware handle and tunnel loops in 3D models. In: ACM SIGGRAPH 2008 Papers, pp. 45:1–45:9. ACM, New York (2008). https://doi.org/10.1145/1399504.1360644

8. Edelsbrunner, H., Letscher, D., Zomorodian, A.: Topological persistence and simplification. Discrete Comput. Geom. **28**(4), 511–533 (2002). https://doi.org/10.1007/s00454-002-2885-2

9. Edelsbrunner, H.: Surface tiling with differential topology. In: Desbrun, M., Pottmann, H. (eds.) Eurographics Symposium on Geometry Processing 2005. The Eurographics Association (2005). https://doi.org/10.2312/SGP/SGP05/009-011

10. Edelsbrunner, H., Harer, J.: Computational Topology: An Introduction. American Mathematical Society, Providence (2010)

11. Ghrist, R., Muhammad, A.: Coverage and hole-detection in sensor networks via homology. In: IPSN 2005: Fourth International Symposium on Information Processing in Sensor Networks, pp. 254–260, April 2005. https://doi.org/10.1109/IPSN.2005.1440933

12. Goodman, J.E., O'Rourke, J. (eds.): Handbook of Discrete and Computational Geometry. CRC Press, Inc., Boca Raton (1997)

13. LeCun, Y., Bottou, L., Bengio, Y., Haffner, P., et al.: Gradient-based learning applied to document recognition. Proc. IEEE **86**(11), 2278–2324 (1998)

14. Lee, H., Kang, H., Chung, M.K., Lee, D.S.: Persistent brain network homology from the perspective of dendrogram. IEEE Trans. Med. Imaging **31**, 2267–2277 (2012)

15. Li, C., Ovsjanikov, M., Chazal, F.: Persistence-based structural recognition. In: 2014 IEEE Conference on Computer Vision and Pattern Recognition, pp. 2003–2010, June 2014. https://doi.org/10.1109/CVPR.2014.257

16. Munkres, J.R.: Elements of Algebraic Topology. Addison Wesley Publishing Company (1984). http://www.worldcat.org/isbn/0201045869

17. Oudot, S.: Persistence theory - from quiver representations to data analysis. In: Mathematical Surveys and Monographs (2015)

18. Perea, J.A., Harer, J.: Sliding windows and persistence: an application of topological methods to signal analysis. Found. Comput. Math. **15**, 799–838 (2015)

19. Silva, V.D., Ghrist, R.: Blind swarms for coverage in 2-D. In: Proceedings of Robotics: Science and Systems, p. 01 (2005)

20. Suckling, J.: The mammographic image analysis society digital mammogram database. Exerpta Medica. International Congress Series 1069, January 1994

Deep Compressed Pneumonia Detection for Low-Power Embedded Devices

Hongjia Li[1]($\boxtimes$), Sheng Lin[1], Ning Liu[1], Caiwen Ding[2], and Yanzhi Wang[1]

[1] Northeastern University, Boston, MA 02115, USA
{li.hongjia,lin.sheng,liu.ning}@husky.neu.edu, yanz.wang@northeastern.edu
[2] University of Connecticut, Storrs, CT 06269, USA
caiwen.ding@uconn.edu

Abstract. Deep neural networks (DNNs) have been expanded into medical fields and triggered the revolution of some medical applications by extracting complex features and achieving high accuracy and performance, etc. On the contrast, the large-scale network brings high requirements of both memory storage and computation resource, especially for portable medical devices and other embedded systems. In this work, we first train a DNN for pneumonia detection using the dataset provided by RSNA Pneumonia Detection Challenge [4]. To overcome hardware limitation for implementing large-scale networks, we develop a systematic structured weight pruning method with filter sparsity, column sparsity and combined sparsity. Experiments show that we can achieve up to 36x compression ratio compared to the original model with 106 layers, while maintaining no accuracy degradation. We evaluate the proposed methods on an embedded low-power device, Jetson TX2, and achieve low power usage and high energy efficiency.

Keywords: Pneumonia detection · YOLO · Structured weight pruning

1 Introduction

There are approximately 450 million people globally (about 7% of the population in the world) suffering from pneumonia, and results in about 4 million deaths per year [9,14]. In the United States, pneumonia accounts for over 500,000 visits to emergency departments [3] and over 50,000 deaths in 2015 [1], keeping the ailment on the list of top 10 causes of death in the country. To accurately diagnose and localize pneumonia, a general diagnostic process requires review of a chest radiograph (CXR) by highly trained specialists and confirmation through clinical history, blood exams and vital symptoms.

To improve the efficiency and reach of diagnostic services, many researchers have extensively studied from medical fields and also computer aided design. In the past years, DNNs have been experiencing a rapid and tremendous progress thanks to the new era of big data. Especially for computer vision problems, deep

© Springer Nature Switzerland AG 2019
L. Zhou et al. (Eds.): LABELS 2019/HAL-MICCAI 2019/CuRIOUS 2019, LNCS 11851, pp. 89–97, 2019.
https://doi.org/10.1007/978-3-030-33642-4_10

learning and large-scale annotated image datasets drastically improved the performances of object recognition, detection and segmentation. Through the training processing based on large-scale datasets, DNNs can rapidly learn the complex features and provide helpful functions of diagnose and localization. Many recent works have discussed medical image detection using large-scale neural networks. Based on Chest X-ray dataset [16], recurrent neural cascade model proposed by [15], CheXNet developed by [10], and Text-Image Embedding network (TieNet) introduced by [17]. Despite the promising results obtained by these works, one of the biggest challenges is that all these networks adopted a deep architecture with multiple layers, leading to a large memory storage and computation resource requirement. These make it difficult to implement large DNN models in portable medical devices and embedded systems [7,8].

In order to deploy DNNs on these embedded devices, DNN model compression techniques such as weight pruning, have been proposed for storage reduction and computation acceleration. Recently, works such as [5,20] have made breakthrough on the weight pruning methods for DNNs while maintaining the network accuracy. However, the network structure and weight storage after pruning become highly irregular and therefore the storage of indexing is non-negligible, which undermines the compression ratio and the performance. Therefore, the structured pruning is proposed to incorporate structured sparsity into the weight pruning algorithm [6,18]. The structured sparsity of DNN introduced by pruning methods is hardware-friendly, and it efficiently improves the evaluation of DNNs on embedded devices.

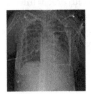 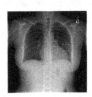 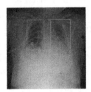 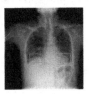

Fig. 1. Examples of pre-processed data. The boxes showed in figure denotes the detected pneumonia.

In this work, we develop a pneumonia detector based on you only look once (YOLO) [11]. We select a dataset provided by RSNA Pneumonia Detection Challenge [4]. In the pre-processing stage, the labeled images are resized to 320×320, along with the corresponding coordinates of bounding boxes, as shown in Fig. 1. YOLOv3 [13] is adopted as the base feature detector with our costumed anchor box priors, due to the speed boost and high average precision. It can achieve detection accuracy of 71.23 mAP. Moreover, in order to enhance the network performance, we utilize training optimizations including learning rate warmup, cosine learning rate decay and mixup training. To further maintain the precision obtained by the 106-layer network, we apply the ADMM-based unified model pruning algorithm on the original model, incorporated with structured sparsity (filter-wise sparsity and column-wise sparsity). Experimental result shows that without accuracy loss, our YOLOv3-based network can be pruned up to 36x.

The number of parameters is reduced from 61.5 M to 1.7 M, which undoubtedly reduces the memory storage and computation resource requirement for embedded systems. To validate our proposed method, we implement our model on Jetson TX2 [2], and it achieves low power usage and high energy efficiency. Therefore, it verifies that our proposed method is very suitable for pneumonia detection with the characteristics of real-time and low-power on portable medical devices.

2 Model Design

2.1 YOLOv3

YOLO is an unified, real-time object detection framework. Compared with other object detection classifiers, YOLO frames object detection as a regression problem to spatially separated bounding boxes and associated class probabilities [11]. Recently, two improved versions of YOLO have been developed, namely YOLO9000 [12] and YOLOv3 [13]. In this work, we adopt YOLOv3 based detector due to its speed boost and high average precision.

YOLOv3 is a fully convolutional network, containing 75 convolutional layers, with skip connections and upsampling layers. The YOLOv3 adopts a convolutional layer with stride 2 as downsampling layer instead of pooling layer. A custom deep architecture Darknet-53 is utilized as the feature extractor since it can achieve a promising performance while with fewer floating point operations and more speedup [13]. In our work, we initialize the weights using a pretrained DarkNet-53 weights based on ImageNet.

YOLOv3 predicts boxes at 3 different scales. For each scale, detection layers that comprised of convolutional layers are constructed, respectively. The last layer predicts a 3D tensor containing bounding box coordinates, object prediction, and class predictions. In our work, the class number is 1 and the number of predicted boxes at each scale is 3, thus the tensor is $N \times N \times [3 * (4 + 1 + 1)]$ for the 4 bounding box offsets, 1 object prediction, and 1 class predictions. YOLOv3 predicts bounding boxes using dimension clusters as anchor boxes. The network predicts 4 coordinates for each bounding box. K-means clustering is adopted to determine our anchor boxes. Same as YOLOv3, we choose 9 clusters and 3 scales. On our data, we modify the 9 clusters as following: $(40 \times 39), (63 \times 49), (48 \times 69), (75 \times 74), (58 \times 102), (83 \times 108), (67 \times 148), (89 \times 154), (94 \times 202)$.

2.2 Training Optimization

Inspired by [19], we absorb several training optimization methods to enhance the network performance. **Learning rate warmup:** Instead of using a too large learning rate directly at the beginning, we use a small learning rate and then smooth back to the initial learning rate. To be specific, we use a gradual warmup strategy, which increases the learning rate from 0 to the original initial learning rate linearly. **Cosine learning rate decay:** For the learning rate decay, a cosine annealing strategy is applied, in which the learning rate gets decreased from the initial value to 0 by the following function: $lr_t = 0.5 * (1 + cos(t\pi/T))lr_0$, where t denotes the current batch and T denotes the total number of batches, and lr_0 is the initial learning rate. **Mixup:** For data augmentation, we adopt mixup method, in which each time we randomly sample two examples (x_i, y_i) and $(x_j.y_j)$. Then a new example is obtained by a weighted linear interpolation of these two examples: $x' = \lambda x_i + (1-\lambda)x_j$, $y' = \lambda y_i + (1-\lambda)y_j$, where $\lambda \in [0,1]$ is a random number drawn from the $Beta(\alpha, \alpha)$ distribution. The new example (x', y') will be used as our training data.

3 Model Compression

3.1 Unified Weight Pruning Algorithm

We develop an unified systematic framework containing three phases: pre-pruning, masked mapping and retraining. The objective of the weight pruning is to minimize the loss function while satisfying the weight constraints, the whole problem is defined as:

$$minimize \ f_{Loss}\big(\{W_i\}_{i=1}^{N}, \{b_i\}_{i=1}^{N}\big), \ subject \ to \ W_i \in \mathcal{S}_i, \ i = 1, \dots, N. \quad (1)$$

where W_i and b_i denotes the sets of weights and biases of the i-th (CONV or FC) layer in an N-layer DNN, respectively. The set $\mathcal{S}_i = \{W_i | card(W_i) \leq \alpha_i\}$ denotes the constraint for weight pruning, and 'card' refers to cardinality. It meets the goal that the number of non-zero elements in W_i is limited by α_i in layer i.

In the pre-pruning phase, we add the ADMM-based regularization on an original DNN model. The regularization is operated by introducing auxiliary variables Z_i's, and dual variables U_i's. In each iteration, while keeping on minimizing network regularized loss, we also reduce the error of Euclidean projection from $W_i^{k+1} + U_i^k$ onto the set $\mathcal{S}_i$. Because under the constraint that α_i is the desired number of weights after pruning in the i-th layer, the Euclidean projection can keep α_i elements in $W_i^{k+1} + U_i^k$ with the largest magnitudes and set the remaining weights to zeros. Then the dual variables U_i is updated as following: $U_i^{k+1} = U_i^k + W_i^{k+1} - Z_i^{k+1}$. In the second phase, with the obtained intermediate W_i solutions, we first perform the Euclidean projection (mapping) to satisfy that at most α_i weights in each layer are non-zero. And then in the retraining phase, the zero weights are gradient masked and non-zero weights are retrained using training sets to restore partial accuracy.

3.2 Structured Pruning

As mentioned before, irregular pruning methods introduce extra storage for index and undermines the compression ratio and the performance. In order to develop an algorithm more friendly on hardware implementation, we incorporate structured pruning with the unified weight pruning algorithm.

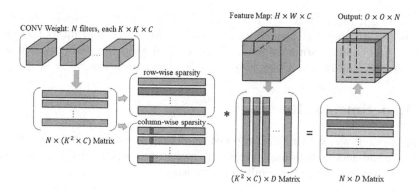

Fig. 2. Examples of GEMM in CONV layer and effect of structured sparsities.

In a typical convolutional layer, there are two structured sparsities: filter-wise sparsity, channel-wise sparsity, and shape-wise sparsity. For fully-connected layers, there are two types: row-wise sparsity and column-wise sparsity. We mainly focus on compressing convolutional layer in our design, since it is the most computationally intensive layer in current DNNs and our model is a fully convolutional network.

During the convolutional computation, the feature map tensor and weights tensor are converted to 2D matrices and performed the general matrix multiplication (GEMM), as shown in Fig. 2. Filter-wise sparsity corresponds to row-wise sparsity, while channel-wise sparsity and shape-wise sparsity correspond to column-wise sparsity. Therefore, filter pruning leads to reducing the number of rows of matrix, and correspondingly, channel and shape pruning result in the reduction of column number. The process of our structured pruning method can be explained as follows.

Filter Pruning. As we mentioned in Eq. 1, the constraint set $\mathcal{S}_i$ here indicates the number of nonzero filters in W_i that is less than a predefined value α_i. To determine the limited number of nonzero filters, we perform $l2\ norm$ on each filter and select the α_i filters with most magnitude and set the remaining as zero.

Column Pruning. In the pre-pruning phase, we prune the convolutional weight by first converting 4D weight tensor into a 2D matrix. Therefore, the constraint set $\mathcal{S}_i$ for column pruning indicates the number of nonzero column in converted W_i that is less than a threshold value. The largest α_i columns evaluated by $l2\ norm$ are kept and the remaining column values are set to zero.

Combined Pruning. To take advantage of utilization in structured pruning on hardware implementation, we propose a approach by combination of these two structured pruning, which decreases the dimension in GEMM while still maintaining a full matrix. We first perform either one type pruning, filter for example. With the filter-pruned model, we first mask the zero filters and then perform the column pruning. In this way, we can keep the desired number of nonzero filter and obtain a higher sparsity on the column-wise.

4   Experimental Results

In this section, we evaluate the proposed model compression technique, starting from original model training, systematic structured weight pruning, and the hardware implementation on embedded device.

4.1   Data Preprocessing

In our project, we use the dataset provided by RSNA Pneumonia Detection Challenge [4]. The dataset is derived from National Institutes of Health Clinical Center for publicly providing the Chest X-Ray dataset [16]. In our experiments, only the labeled images are selected, loaded from Digital Imaging and Communications in Medicine (DICOM) image format and resized into 320×320 from the original 1024×1024. The corresponding coordinates are also re-calculated from the original size. The whole dataset contains 6,002 images, of which 5,400 are considered as our training dataset and the remaining 602 are test dataset.

4.2   Model Training

We apply the weight pruning method and train the pneumonia detector on Nvidia GeForce GTX2080 using Pytorch. During the training, we warmup our learning rate from 10^{-5} to our initial learning rate 10^{-3} during the first epoch. In the rest epochs, the learning rate decreased from 10^{-3} to 4^{-8} using the cosine function. The α for the *Beta* distribution in data mixup is 0.2.

4.3   Model Evaluation

To evaluate the performance of the model, we use mean average precision (mAP) at different intersection over union (IoU) thresholds. The metric sweeps over a range of IoU thresholds, at each point calculating an average precision value. The threshold values range from 0.4 to 0.75 with a step size of 0.05: (0.4, 0.45, 0.5, 0.55, 0.6, 0.65, 0.7, 0.75). To be specific, if we use 0.5 as the threshold, only when IoU is greater than 0.5 the object can be considered as detected. The result of original model is listed on the first row in Table 1 under different IoU thresholds. When IoU threshold is 0.5, we can achieve detection accuracy of 71.23 mAP.

Next, the unified structured weight pruning method is applied on filter pruning, column pruning and combined pruning, respectively. The detailed evaluation results of models with various prune ratio are shown in Table 1. Without accuracy loss, the prune ratio can be increased up to 36x. For this model, we prune 3.56x filters and 9.68x columns. The size of model parameters is reduced from

61.5 M to 1.7 M, which results the model storage saved from 246.4 MB to 6.84 MB. The original floating point operations (FLOPs) is 38.63 Bn. In total, the FLOPs can be significantly reduced to 1.32 Bn. In this way, not only the requirement of memory storage and computation resource decreased, but also facilitate acceleration on embedded devices.

Table 1. Localization accuracy (mAP) using IoU where T(IoU) = 0.4, 0.45, 0.5, 0.55, 0.6, 0.65, 0.7, 0.75.

T(IoU)		0.4	0.45	**0.5**	0.55	0.6	0.65	0.7	0.75
Original model		81.2	76.3	**71.2**	63.4	54.7	42.3	30.7	19.1
Filter pruned	11.55x	81.4	75.9	**71.5**	63.8	53.0	40.9	29.7	17.9
	16.26x	80.6	76.2	**71.2**	62.5	53.6	42.3	30.0	18.7
	19.33x	80.7	76.1	**71.1**	62.3	52.9	41.2	30.0	18.6
Column pruned	11.60x	81.2	76.9	**71.9**	64.5	53.3	41.8	29.8	18.4
	16.36x	80.7	76.0	**71.3**	64.1	55.9	41.5	28.4	19.1
	19.55x	80.6	76.1	**71.0**	63.7	53.5	42.3	29.7	18.7
Combined pruned	**36.02x**	**81.2**	**76.3**	71.0	**63.5**	**53.4**	**42.8**	**31.2**	**19.3**
	51.97x	81.0	76.0	**70.6**	62.8	53.0	41.7	29.0	18.3

4.4 Hardware Implementation

To validate our method on the embedded low-power devices, we implement our pruned model on Jetson TX2, which is considered as the fastest, most power-efficient embedded AI computing device [2]. It's built by a 256-core NVIDIA Pascal-family GPU and the memory is 8 GB with 59.7 GB/s bandwidth. The power consumption of our model is 7.3 W and the energy efficiency is 0.69 IPS/W. The low power usage and high energy efficiency show a high feasibility and compatibility of our weight pruning method on DNN for low-power real-world devices.

5 Conclusion

In this work, we developed a YOLOv3-based detector for pneumonia detection with 71.23 mAP. In order to reduce the storage memory and computational resource requirement by the 106-layer fully convolution network, we applied a systematic structured weight pruning method on filter sparsity, column sparsity and combined sparsity. Without accuracy loss, the prune ratio can achieve up to 36x, which reduce the model size from 61.5 M to 1.7 M. To validate our method on the real-world low-power device, we implemented and evaluated our model on Jetson TX2, which resulted a low power usage and high energy efficiency.

References

1. Deaths: Final data for 2015. supplemental tables. https://www.cdc.gov/nchs/data/nvsr/nvsr66/nvsr66_06_tables.pdf. Accessed 24 May 2019
2. Jetson tx2 module. https://developer.nvidia.com/embedded/buy/jetson-tx2
3. National ambulatory medical care survey: 2015 emergency department summary tables. https://www.cdc.gov/nchs/data/nhamcs/web_tables/2015_ed_web_tables.pdf. Accessed 24 May 2019
4. Rsna pneumonia detection challenge (2018). https://www.kaggle.com/c/rsna-pneumonia-detection-challenge/overview
5. Han, S., Mao, H., Dally, W.J.: Deep compression: Compressing deep neural networks with pruning, trained quantization and huffman coding. arXiv preprint arXiv:1510.00149 (2015)
6. He, Y., Zhang, X., Sun, J.: Channel pruning for accelerating very deep neural networks. In: International Conference on Computer Vision (ICCV), vol. 2 (2017)
7. Li, H., et al.: ADMM-based weight pruning for real-time deep learning acceleration on mobile devices. In: Proceedings of the 2019 on Great Lakes Symposium on VLSI, pp. 501–506. ACM (2019)
8. Lin, S., et al.: FFT-based deep learning deployment in embedded systems. In: 2018 Design, Automation & Test in Europe Conference & Exhibition (DATE), pp. 1045–1050. IEEE (2018)
9. Lodha, R., Kabra, S.K., Pandey, R.M.: Antibiotics for community-acquired pneumonia in children. Cochrane Database Syst. Rev. (6) (2013)
10. Rajpurkar, P., et al.: Chexnet: radiologist-level pneumonia detection on Chest X-rays with deep learning. arXiv preprint arXiv:1711.05225 (2017)
11. Redmon, J., Divvala, S., Girshick, R., Farhadi, A.: You only look once: unified, real-time object detection. In: Proceedings of the IEEE Conference on Computer Vision and Pattern Recognition, pp. 779–788 (2016)
12. Redmon, J., Farhadi, A.: YOLO9000: better, faster, stronger. In: Proceedings of the IEEE Conference on Computer Vision and Pattern Recognition, pp. 7263–7271 (2017)
13. Redmon, J., Farhadi, A.: YOLOv3: an incremental improvement. arXiv preprint arXiv:1804.02767 (2018)
14. Ruuskanen, O., Lahti, E., Jennings, L.C., Murdoch, D.R.: Viral pneumonia. Lancet **377**(9773), 1264–1275 (2011)
15. Shin, H.C., Roberts, K., Lu, L., Demner-Fushman, D., Yao, J., Summers, R.M.: Learning to read chest x-rays: recurrent neural cascade model for automated image annotation. In: Proceedings of the IEEE Conference on Computer Vision and Pattern Recognition, pp. 2497–2506 (2016)
16. Wang, X., Peng, Y., Lu, L., Lu, Z., Bagheri, M., Summers, R.M.: Chestx-ray8: hospital-scale chest x-ray database and benchmarks on weakly-supervised classification and localization of common thorax diseases. In: Proceedings of the IEEE Conference on Computer Vision and Pattern Recognition, pp. 2097–2106 (2017)
17. Wang, X., Peng, Y., Lu, L., Lu, Z., Summers, R.M.: TieNet: text-image embedding network for common thorax disease classification and reporting in chest x-rays. In: Proceedings of the IEEE Conference on Computer Vision and Pattern Recognition, pp. 9049–9058 (2018)
18. Wen, W., Wu, C., Wang, Y., Chen, Y., Li, H.: Learning structured sparsity in deep neural networks. In: Advances in Neural Information Processing Systems, pp. 2074–2082 (2016)

19. Xie, J., He, T., Zhang, Z., Zhang, H., Zhang, Z., Li, M.: Bag of tricks for image classification with convolutional neural networks. arXiv preprint arXiv:1812.01187 (2018)
20. Zhang, T., et al.: A systematic DNN weight pruning framework using alternating direction method of multipliers. arXiv preprint arXiv:1804.03294 (2018)

D3MC: A Reinforcement Learning Based Data-Driven Dyna Model Compression

Jiahui Guan, Ravi Soni, Dibyajyoti Pati, Gopal Avinash,
and V. Ratna Saripalli[✉]

GE Healthcare, San Ramon, CA, USA
Ratna.Saripalli@ge.com

Abstract. Artificial intelligence (AI)-driven medical devices have created a new excitement in healthcare sector. While deeper and wider neural networks are designed for complex healthcare applications, model compression can be an effective way to deploy networks on medical devices that often have hardware and speed constraints. Most state-of-the-art model compression techniques require a resource centric manual process that explores a large model architecture space to find a trade-off solution between model size and accuracy. Recently, reinforcement learning (RL) approaches are proposed to automate such a hand-crafted process. However, most RL model compression algorithms are model-free that require longer time with no assumptions of the model. On the contrary, model-based (MB) approaches are data driven; have faster convergence but are sensitive to the bias in the model. In this paper, we develop data-driven dyna model compression (D3MC) algorithm that integrates model-based and model-free RL approaches. We evaluate our algorithm on a variety of imaging data from dermoscopy to X-ray on different popular and public model architectures. Compared to model-free RL approaches, our approach achieves faster convergence; exhibits better generalization across different data sets; and preserves comparable model performance.

Keywords: Model compression · Reinforcement learning · Dyna · Automation

1 Introduction

Medical devices such as X-ray, MR, CT and Ultrasound need deep neural networks (DNN) to bring down operational costs and improve performance. Reducing the size of DNNs is pivotal for maximizing the benefits of medical devices with limited computational resources. Model compression techniques, to reduce the size of DNNs, comes with a trade-off between compression and performance. Randomly reducing a network may adversely affect the model performance.

J. Guan and R. Soni—Equal contribution.

© Springer Nature Switzerland AG 2019
L. Zhou et al. (Eds.): LABELS 2019/HAL-MICCAI 2019/CuRIOUS 2019, LNCS 11851, pp. 98–105, 2019.
https://doi.org/10.1007/978-3-030-33642-4_11

Over the past years, researchers have developed techniques that utilize a hand-designed smaller network that can achieve similar performance as the original network. Hand-designed approaches require extensive manual effort from a domain expert and might not be the optimal solution. Recently there has been a considerable amount of work towards automation of model compression using reinforcement learning (RL). Most of these RL techniques are model-free (MF), without any assumptions of the model or samples. Such approaches are often flexible and learn complex policies effectively, but their global convergence requires large number of trials. On the contrary, model-based (MB) techniques have strong theoretical basis; generalize better; and, usually converge faster [2]. Though practically efficient, MB approaches suffer from bias sensitivity and model selection difficulty.

In this paper, we propose a data-driven dyna model compression (D3MC) framework to bridge the gap between MB and MF approaches. Compared to MF methods, our hybrid approach significantly reduces the training time. We use a greedy α weight between MF and MB, that can be parametrized to decrease over time. The reward prediction from the MB component can be generalized across different data sets for any given network architecture. To the best of our knowledge, this is the first hybrid reinforcement learning (RL) based neural network compression method applied in medical imaging domain. We benchmarked our methods on public health data sets. Our experimental results show that D3MC requires much less training time while maintaining similar model performance.

Related Work: There are several conventional approaches to compress a neural network to a hand-crafted model such as pruning [6], quantization [7] and knowledge distillation [4]. Pruning-based approaches remove redundant weights and only keep weights that contributes to the final output. Quantization approach constrains the inputs resulting in reduced networks. Knowledge distillation approach requires training a given smaller network with respect to the input teacher network so that the performance of two models are comparable [4]. However, all of those methods require non-trivial manual selections. Recently, RL approaches have been developed to automate the network compression. Ashok et al. [1] proposed N2N learning and He et al. [3] used AMC engine to reduce neural network sizes. However, most of them are MF approaches, which are time-consuming requiring RL agent to explore a large architecture space.

Compared to MF methods, MB approaches require much less training time but underlying dynamics is difficult to estimate. Dyna architecture [8] combines MF and MB by integrating planning, acting and learning. However, the original paper on dyna structure uses Q-table, which is inefficient for large problem space [8]. Instead, we use a functional approximation approach that is more robust.

The main contributions of the paper include (1) proposing a new model compression algorithm that combines MB and MF approaches, (2) the first of its kind in the applications on medical imaging, (3) applying RL compression methods on complex network architectures such as Inception-v3 that are most commonly used in imaging classification and (4) layer removal pattern analysis across different datasets for similar network architectures.

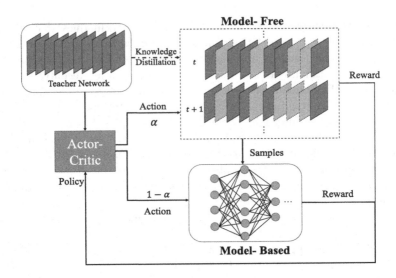

Fig. 1. The workflow of reinforcement learning training process of D3MC.

2 Methods

Our proposed D3MC is analogous to dyna architecture where the MB component is built from the data generated from the MF component as sown in Fig. 1. We consider the standard RL setting in our D3MC pipeline, that is, an agent interacts with an environment over a number of time steps or trials. At each time step t, the agent receives a state s_t, which is a reduced student network, and selects an action a_t based on its policy π. The policy π is a mapping from s_t to a_t. a_t is a list of binary actions (0 to keep, 1 to remove) corresponding to each layer in the network. The agent then receives the next state s_{t+1} as well as a reward r_t. This iterative process continues for N time steps, where N is sufficiently large that the reward converges (Algorithm 1). The detailed setting of RL framework is as follows:

Environment: Teacher network architectures. The environment accepts a list of layers to be removed from the RL agent.

State: All possible reduced student network architectures derived from the teacher model.

Action: Remove layer or not.

Agent: Actor-Critic based agent.

Optimization: Under actor-critic architecture, the policy is directly parameterized $\pi(a|s; \theta)$. To optimize θ, we use REINFORCE family of policy gradient algorithm [11] that updates θ at each time step t with respect to its gradient ascent on $E[R_t]$. Given that $\nabla_\theta \log \pi(a_t|s_t; \theta) R_t$ is an unbiased estimator of $\nabla_\theta E(R_t)$ and subtracting a baseline can reduce its variances, we update the policy parameters θ in the direction of

$$\nabla_\theta J(\theta) = \nabla_\theta \log \pi(a_t|s_t; \theta)(R_t - b_t(s_t)) \tag{1}$$

Algorithm 1. Algorithm of D3MC

1: $s_0 \leftarrow$ Teacher model
2: **for** $i = 1, ...N$ **do**
3:    **for** $t = 1, ..L_1$ **do**
4:       $a_t \sim \pi_{\text{remove}}(s_{t-1}; \theta_{\text{remove},i-1})$
5:       $s_t \leftarrow T(s_{t-1}, a_t)$
6:       Sample $u^* \sim \text{Unifom}(0, 1)$
7:       **if** $u^* > \alpha$ **then** $\triangleright$ Model-Free
8:          $R \leftarrow r(s_{L_1})$
9:       **else** $\triangleright$ Model-Based
10:          $R \leftarrow f(a_t, l, k, ks, s, p, n)$
11:    $\theta_{\text{remove},i} \leftarrow \nabla_{\theta_{\text{remove},i-1}} J(\theta_{\text{remove},i-1})$
12: **Output:** Student model.

We use a learned estimate of the value function $V^\pi(s_t)$, which is the critic, as the baseline b_t.

The MB component is a dense neural network to predict the reward (Fig. 1). We use α to weigh MF and MB components (where $\alpha \in [0, 1]$). As MB component generalizes, we decay α to reduce MF dependency.

Model-Free Reward: MF component learns an effective policy from rewards alone. Reward is a combination of compression and accuracy ratio. In this paper, we define MF reward [1] as: $R = C(2 - C) \cdot \dfrac{\text{Acc}_{\text{student}}}{\text{Acc}_{\text{teacher}}}$.

where $C \in [0, 1)$ is the compression ratio defined as $C = 1 - \dfrac{\#\text{param}_{\text{student}}}{\#\text{param}_{\text{teacher}}}$.
Acc is the accuracy produced by the model.

Model-Based Reward: MB reward value is computed as a function of layer description as shown in Eq. 2 using a six-layer dense deep neural network.

$$R = f(x_t) \tag{2}$$

where $x_t = (a_t, l, k, ks, s, p, n)$. $a_t \in \{0, 1\}_{(L_1-1) \times 1}$ is the action list, l is the layer type, k is the number of kernels, ks is the kernel size, s is stride, p is padding and n is trainable parameters. The MB training loss is mean squared error (MSE) and we use cross-validation to evaluate the model. Since there are no assumed distributions such as Gaussian, this function f is driven by the data, which is more representative of the heuristic data structure.

3 Experiments and Results

Datasets: We demonstrated our D3MC algorithm on general images CIFAR-10, chest X-ray Pneumothorax (PTX), chest X-ray NLM Frontal, and dermatoscopis images Ham10k for classification problems. The CIFAR-10 dataset [5] consists of 10 classes of objects and is divided into 50,000 train and 10,000 test images (32 × 32 pixels). The datasets of PTX are chest X-ray images with pneumothorax disease that were released by NIH Clinical Center [10]. The scanned images consist more than 30,000 patients. The National Library of Medicine (NLM) frontal dataset were used as a binary classification to group chest X-ray images into frontal or non-frontal position views [12]. There are approximately 8300 images of size 256 × 256. We also evaluated Human Against Machine with 10000 training images (Ham10k) [9] that contains 10015 dermatoscopic images to classify pigmented skin lesions.

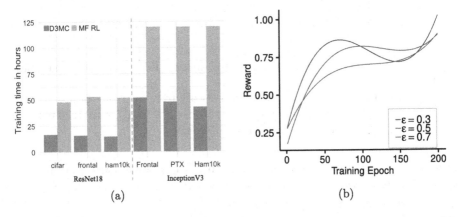

Fig. 2. Training time comparison and α exploration. (a) Training time in hours. (b) D3MC rewards of different values of α. Decreasing α gives faster convergence.

Training Time Comparison: We evaluated our method with automated model compression techniques for fair comparison. All the experiments were trained on Tesla V100 GPUs. We benchmarked our D3MC to MF RL on ResNet-18 and Inception-v3. In the RL training, we used ADAM optimizer with a learning rate 0.001. Based on our experiments, α of 0.3 for ResNet-18 and 0.5 for Inception-v3 gave the best performance. We set the same training steps for MF RL and D3MC to avoid any biases.

The training time comparison is visualized in Fig. 2(a). The training time of D3MC is significantly less on both ResNet-18 and Inception-v3 architectures compared to MF RL. For example, it took over 120 h (5 days) to train Inception-v3 using MF only approach while our D3MC shortened it approximately by 60% of the time to 2 days. It is clear that our D3MC is more efficient than MF RL approaches.

Model Compression Performance: Our experimental results show comparable model performance. Table 1 illustrates the network compression ratio and model accuracy of the optimal compressed networks. Both MF RL and D3MC

Table 1. Summary of top reward models' results.

Architecture	Training data	Method	MB training data	Training time (hrs)	Compression ratio	Teacher Acc.	Δ Acc.
ResNet - 18	Cifar10	Model-Free	–	48	47.68%	86.4%	2.94%
		D3MC	Cifar10	**17**	50.0%	84.4%	2.75%
	Frontal	Model-Free	–	53	94.3%	99.5%	0.3%
		D3MC	Cifar10	**16**	78.0%	99.0%	0.4%
	Ham10k	Model-Free	–	52	65.41%	82.55%	3.29%
		D3MC	Cifar10 +Frontal	**14.8**	76.27%	81.47%	2.073%
Inception - v3	Frontal	Model-Free	–	120	60.7%	99.6%	0.28%
		D3MC	Frontal	**48**	58.96%	99.59%	0.21%
	PTX	Model-Free	–	120	36.4%	82.2%	1.96%
		D3MC	Frontal	**52**	52.3%	81.99%	2.85%
	Ham10k	Model-Free	–	83	47.42%	83.69%	3.16%
		D3MC	Frontal +PTX	**27**	46.26%	81.99%	3.042%

heavily reduced the size of ResNet-18 and Inception-v3, with minimal impact to model performance. The differences between MF RL and D3MC are very small compared to the teacher accuracy. With slight loss of compression ratio and model accuracy, D3MC provides a significant gain of training time (shown in the last column in Table 1) and better generalization across different data sets.

Analysis of α: To better understand the impact of α, we analyzed the reward with different values of α in Fig. 2(b). After fitting the rewards with B-spline, we observed that decreasing α resulted in faster convergence.

Layer Removal Pattern: We investigated the layer removal patterns and their variations among different datasets. In Fig. 3, the two layers with highest number of parameters (almost 1.5 million) have been removed in all three students with almost negligible reduction in performance. The common removed layers across datasets weigh approximately 36% of original Inception-v3 teacher network. We further conducted paired Wilcoxon rank significance test of the layer removal across the data sets. We fail to reject the null hypothesis that the paired three groups are identical with p-values 0.72 (PTX vs Ham10k), 0.93 (Frontal vs PTX) and 0.74 (Frontal vs Ham10k). This observation suggests that there is a common layer removal pattern across the tested healthcare datasets.

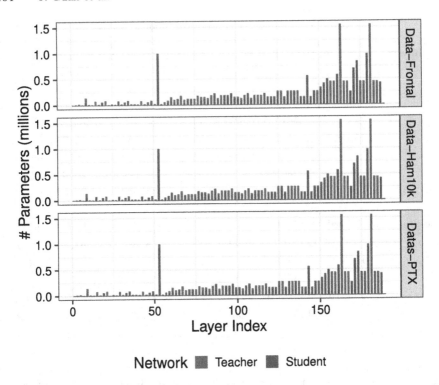

Fig. 3. The layer removal pattern of Inception-v3 on frontal, ham10k and PTX datasets. The layers with non-zero parameters of the top student network (green) are overlaid on the teacher network (red). (Color figure online)

4   Discussion and Conclusion

In this paper, we introduced D3MC framework that integrates the model-based and model-free approaches to significantly reduce RL training time and output optimally compressed models. We show that our method performs well on a variety of healthcare data sets and model architectures. D3MC framework has improved our compression pipeline efficiency and cutdown the training time by over 65%. We demonstrated that our RL agent generalizes across different datasets for a given architecture and compresses InceptionV3 network over 55% while maintaining comparable model performance. The optimal compressed model can further be fine-tuned as part of post-processing to achieve even better performance.

In order to avoid potential overfitting, we plan to incorporate early stopping in our RL algorithm. One idea is to adopt a compression ratio and/or accuracy constraint. Because healthcare projects have different requirements in terms of model sizes and accuracies, such constraints can be used as a terminal state for early stopping. Additionally, we will explore further individual network components that drive compression factors to improve the efficiency and generalization of the RL agent across different network architectures. We are in the process of exploring compression techniques for segmentation and other machine learning patterns.

In conclusion, to build smart medical devices there is a need for efficient model compression techniques. In order to address this need, we have introduced D3MC framework to simultaneously reduce training time and improve compression while maintaining performance across healthcare datasets. Our experiments have shown promising results on two standard networks used for classification.

Acknowledgments. We thank Amazon Sagemaker RL team for collaborating with us and providing the network model compression example.

References

1. Ashok, A., Rhinehart, N., Beainy, F., Kitani, K.M.: N2N learning: Network to network compression via policy gradient reinforcement learning. arXiv preprint arXiv:1709.06030 (2017)
2. Bansal, S., Calandra, R., Chua, K., Levine, S., Tomlin, C.: MBMF: Model-based priors for model-free reinforcement learning. arXiv preprint arXiv:1709.03153 (2017)
3. He, Y., Lin, J., Liu, Z., Wang, H., Li, L.-J., Han, S.: AMC: AutoML for model compression and acceleration on mobile devices. In: Ferrari, V., Hebert, M., Sminchisescu, C., Weiss, Y. (eds.) ECCV 2018. LNCS, vol. 11211, pp. 815–832. Springer, Cham (2018). https://doi.org/10.1007/978-3-030-01234-2_48
4. Hinton, G., Vinyals, O., Dean, J.: Distilling the knowledge in a neural network. arXiv preprint arXiv:1503.02531 (2015)
5. Krizhevsky, A., Hinton, G.: Learning multiple layers of features from tiny images. Technical report, Citeseer (2009)
6. Polyak, A., Wolf, L.: Channel-level acceleration of deep face representations. IEEE Access **3**, 2163–2175 (2015)
7. Rastegari, M., Ordonez, V., Redmon, J., Farhadi, A.: XNOR-Net: ImageNet classification using binary convolutional neural networks. In: Leibe, B., Matas, J., Sebe, N., Welling, M. (eds.) ECCV 2016. LNCS, vol. 9908, pp. 525–542. Springer, Cham (2016). https://doi.org/10.1007/978-3-319-46493-0_32
8. Sutton, R.S., Szepesvári, C., Geramifard, A., Bowling, M.P.: Dyna-style planning with linear function approximation and prioritized sweeping. arXiv preprint arXiv:1206.3285 (2012)
9. Tschandl, P., Rosendahl, C., Kittler, H.: The ham10000 dataset, a large collection of multi-source dermatoscopic images of common pigmented skin lesions. Sci. Data **5**, 180161 (2018)
10. Wang, X., Peng, Y., Lu, L., Lu, Z., Bagheri, M., Summers, R.M.: ChestX-ray8: hospital-scale chest x-ray database and benchmarks on weakly-supervised classification and localization of common thorax diseases. In: 2017 IEEE Conference on Computer Vision and Pattern Recognition (CVPR), pp. 3462–3471. IEEE (2017)
11. Williams, R.J.: Simple statistical gradient-following algorithms for connectionist reinforcement learning. Mach. Learn. **8**(3–4), 229–256 (1992)
12. Xue, Z., et al.: Chest x-ray image view classification. In: 2015 IEEE 28th International Symposium on Computer-Based Medical Systems (CBMS), pp. 66–71. IEEE (2015)

An Analytical Method of Automatic Alignment for Electron Tomography

Shuang Wen[✉] and Guojie Luo[✉]

Center for Energy-efficient Computing and Applications,
Peking University, Beijing 100871, China
{wenshuang,gluo}@pku.edu.cn
http://ceca.pku.edu.cn

Abstract. In the imaging process for nanometer-scale electron tomography, misalignment between the actual projection parameters and the theoretical ones is inevitable due to mechanical precision of the instrument. Effective alignment remains a challenge. Currently, marker-based alignment approaches complicate the sample preparation process and worsen the sample shrinking issue. Marker-free approaches suffer from either low accuracy or long computation time.

In this paper, we formulate an analytical problem for marker-free alignment by minimizing the reprojection error. The reprojection error involves the projection operator, which is a complicated functional with the projection parameters as the variables. To solve this optimization problem, we derive a gradient-based approach by decomposing the original problem with auxiliary parameters and by linearizing a subproblem with Taylor expansion. The approach is computational friendly, especially when comparing to an exhaustively parameter tuning approach in previous practice. The results show that our method is capable of accurate alignment without fiducial markers and obtains a 16.7× speedup over the existing exhaustive approach, which makes fine reconstruction of ROI almost instantly ready after data collection. A preliminary FPGA design for the method's bottleneck process shows 6.6× speed-up over well-optimized GPU program.

Keywords: Electron tomography · Automatic alignment · Functional optimization

1 Introduction

Electron tomography (ET), a technique combining transmission electron microscopy (TEM) and computed tomography, is now widely used for acquiring high-resolution 3D structures of biological samples. To obtain the 3D structures, it is critical to reconstruct the region of interest (ROI) from projection images provided by the TEM microscope. These projection images are usually collected

© Springer Nature Switzerland AG 2019
L. Zhou et al. (Eds.): LABELS 2019/HAL-MICCAI 2019/CuRIOUS 2019, LNCS 11851, pp. 106–114, 2019.
https://doi.org/10.1007/978-3-030-33642-4_12

according to specific regulations called tilt geometries. A tilt geometry decides the position and attitude of a series of projection images (tilt series) for ET reconstruction.

We perform ET reconstruction given the theoretical tilt geometry and the tilt series. However, due to high magnification and low mechanical accuracy, unexpected drift and rotation of ROI happen during the image collection process. Therefore, alignment is needed for high-quality reconstruction results.

There are mainly two types of alignment methods, marker-based alignment and marker-free alignment. Fiducial marker-based alignment approaches [8,10] use high-contrast markers, such as gold beads, embedded in a sample to determine the position and attitude of the tilt series. However, this type of method is not always available, since it is difficult or impossible to embed enough fiducial markers in the ROI sometimes. Besides, the selection of marker detection algorithms is data-dependent [11], which also limits the usability of the marker-based approaches.

Marker-free alignment approaches require no embedded fiducial markers. And these methods can be further categorized into cross-correlation and feature-based methods. Guckenberger [2] brought up cross-correlation alignment method which determines the common origin of tilt series by comparing the cross-correlation coefficient. But this method is bothered by errors accumulating along with alignment going on. For this problem, Winkler and Taylor [13] proposed a method combining cross-correlation and reconstruction-reprojection to compensate accumulated errors, which is still widely used. This method will be mention below as naive exhaustive search (NES) method On the other hand, feature-based methods make use of image features as markers to do the alignment. Feature-based methods is often less time-consuming [3] but need specific detectors for different kind of datasets [11], which damages its universality.

To overcome these problems, the method presented in this paper is developed for reconstructing specimens without fiducial markers and apparent local features. Inspired by Houben and Sadan [5], method is mainly composed of a coarse alignment process by cross-correlation and a refinement process based on minimization of reprojection error. The former coarse alignment is used to provide the latter process with an initial value. The following refinement process further improves the alignment accuracy. With both procedures, we grantee the algorithm with both efficiency and accuracy. Compared with other methods, our method does not depend on fiducial markers or image features. Through reconstruction and reprojection process, both projection space and real space information are made full use of, which makes our method free from accumulated correlation errors that happen in the cross-correlation method. Compared with the iterative reconstruction-reprojection method brought up by Winkler and Taylor [13], as experimental results show, less iteration number needed and fewer operations within one iteration make our method much efficient. The experiment on a conical-tilt dataset shows our method's comparable accuracy and 16.7× efficiency compared with similar marker-free method. For the method's bottleneck process, a preliminary FPGA design shows 6.6× speed-up over a well-optimized GPU program.

2   Automatic Alignment Problem

We reconstruct the 3-D image of a specimen from a collection of 2-D TEM images (projections) using electron tomography. The process is determined by a set of parameters in θ. For a fixed tilt angle, we collect N projections of the specimen at configuration $\theta = (\theta_1, \theta_2, \cdots, \theta_N)$. The i-th projection is determined by a 5-tuple $\theta_i = (\alpha_i, \beta_i, \gamma_i, x_i, y_i)$, where the ROI center of the specimen is projected at coordinate (x_i, y_i), and α_i, β_i and γ_i are the yaw, pitch, and roll angles of the specimen, respectively.

Ideally, the 5-tuple of each projection is known at prior. Using an automatic, a semi-automatic, or a manual controller, we take TEM images at certain angles by rotating the specimen along its normal with a fixed tilt. The specimen's ideal posture at certain configuration is as shown in Fig. 1.

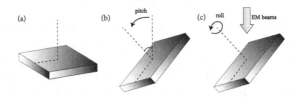

Fig. 1. (a) Original specimen. (b) Tilt specimen with a fixed pitch. (c) A series of tilt specimen with various roll angles.

At each angle, we obtain the corresponding yaw, pitch, and roll angles, and we shift, align, and refocus the ROI center before taking a TEM image.

However, due to the intrinsic random and system errors of the instrument (e.g., the controller, the motor, and the tray), the actual configuration $\theta_i^* = (\alpha_i^* + \epsilon_{\alpha_i}, \beta_i^* + \epsilon_{\beta_i}, \gamma_i^* + \epsilon_{\gamma_i}, x_i^* + \epsilon_{x_i}, y_i^* + \epsilon_{y_i})$ is different from the ideal configuration $\tilde{\theta}_i = (\alpha_i^*, \beta_i^*, \gamma_i^*, x_i^*, y_i^*)$.

Assuming f^* is the unobservable 3-D image, the TEM imaging process can be described using the projection operator $\mathcal{R}(\theta^*) = (\mathcal{R}(\theta_1^*), \mathcal{R}(\theta_2^*), \cdots, \mathcal{R}(\theta_N^*))$. And the projection data $g = \mathcal{R}(\theta^*)f^* = (g_1, g_2, \cdots, g_N)$ consists of a set of 2-D TEM images, the i-th of which is $g_i = \mathcal{R}(\theta_i^*)$.

If we use the mistakenly-believed ideal configuration $\tilde{\theta}$ to reconstruct the 3-D image by solving for $\operatorname{argmin}_f \|\mathcal{R}(\tilde{\theta})f - g\|^2$, it will always generate inaccurate results, since $\mathcal{R}(\tilde{\theta})f^* \neq g = \mathcal{R}(\theta^*)f^*$. Therefore, we propose the automatic correction problem to recover the actual configuration θ^* for a high-quality electron tomography, so that we can avoid the quality degradation due to using the mistakenly-believed ideal configuration $\tilde{\theta}$ during image reconstruction. For convenience consideration, we mark $\operatorname{argmin}_f \|\mathcal{R}(\tilde{\theta})f - g\|^2$ with $\mathcal{S}(\theta, g)$.

We formulate automatic correction as a functional optimization problem,

$$\min_{\theta} \quad \|\mathcal{R}(\theta)f(\theta) - g\|^2$$
$$\text{where } f(\theta) = \operatorname*{argmin}_{f} \|\mathcal{R}(\theta)f - g\|^2. \tag{1}$$

The parameterized operator (functional) $\mathcal{R}(\theta)$ models how the projection data g is acquired, and the image $f(\theta)$ is reconstructed at the guess of projection configuration θ.

Apparently, the actual configuration θ^* is an exact solution to this problem, such that $||\mathcal{R}(\theta^*)f(\theta^*) - g|| = ||\mathcal{R}(\theta^*)f^* - g|| = 0$. By solving the automatic correction problem to recover an estimate of the actual configuration $\hat{\theta}$, we expect to "correct" the mistakenly-believed ideal $\tilde{\theta}$, so that $||\mathcal{R}(\hat{\theta})f(\hat{\theta}) - g|| < ||\mathcal{R}(\tilde{\theta})f(\tilde{\theta}) - g||$, if not $||\mathcal{R}(\hat{\theta})f(\hat{\theta}) - g|| = 0$.

3   Automatic Alignment Methods

3.1   Naive Exhaustive Search

The basic idea of naive exhaustive search is to examine the neighborhood of known parameters in the solution space and find the best solution in this neighborhood by comparing the values of the objective function. Taking a projection series with 72 projections and each projection with 5 configuration parameters for example, the solution space dimension is $72 \times 5 = 360$. A search in 360-dimension space requires objective function $\mathcal{S}$ and $\mathcal{R}$ calculated large amount of times.

3.2   Analytical Optimization

The key of our method is the optimize of Eq. (1) using gradient descent method. This process involves computing the gradients $\nabla_\theta \mathcal{R}(\theta)$ and $\nabla_\theta f(\theta)$. The latter one is relatively difficult to write down the analytical form. To use the gradient descent method, we reformulate Eq. (1) into the following problem by introducing the auxiliary varaible $\bar{\theta}$,

$$\min_{\theta, \bar{\theta}} \quad \left\|\mathcal{R}(\theta)f(\bar{\theta}) - g\right\|^2 \quad \text{s.t.} \bar{\theta} = \theta$$
$$\text{where } f(\bar{\theta}) = \operatorname{argmin}_f \left\|\mathcal{R}(\bar{\theta})f - g\right\|^2 . \tag{2}$$

And we apply a hybrid approach of block descent and gradient projection to solve this reformulated problem. And our algorithm is outlined as below,

Step 0. Start from $k = 0$ with initial guess $\theta^{(0)} = \bar{\theta}^{(0)} = \tilde{\theta}$;
Step 1. Solve $f^{(k)} = \operatorname{argmin}_f ||\mathcal{R}(\bar{\theta}^{(k)})f - g||^2$;
Step 2. Solve $\theta^{(k+1)} = \operatorname{argmin}_\theta ||\mathcal{R}(\theta)f^{(k)} - g||^2$;
Step 3. Update $\bar{\theta}^{(k+1)} = \theta^{(k+1)}$;
Step 4. If not converged, Set $k = k + 1$ and **Goto** Step 1.

The subproblem in Step 1 is the conventional image reconstruction problem for electron tomography. Weighted back-projection is one of the feasible methods.

We solve the subproblem in Step 2 using linearization. It is natural to start with the initial solution $\theta^{(k)}$. We then perform a Taylor expansion at $\theta^{(k)}$ and derive $\mathcal{R}(\theta^{(k)} + \Delta\theta)f^{(k)} = (\mathcal{R}f^{(k)})(\theta^{(k)} + \Delta\theta) \approx (\mathcal{R}f^{(k)})$

$(\theta^{(k)}) + \nabla_\theta(\mathcal{R}f^{(k)})(\theta^{(k)})\Delta\theta$. After solving $\Delta\theta^{(k)} = \text{argmin}_{\Delta\theta}||(\mathcal{R}f^{(k)})(\theta^{(k)}) + \nabla_\theta(\mathcal{R}f^{(k)})(\theta^{(k)})\Delta\theta - g||^2$ by least squares, we update $\theta^{(k+1)} = \theta^{(k)} + \Delta\theta^{(k)}$.

According to the definition of operator $\mathcal{R}$, integration form of $\nabla_\theta(\mathcal{R}f^{(k)})$ $(\theta^{(k)})$ can be expressed by

$$\nabla_\theta(\mathcal{R}f^{(k)})(\theta^{(k)}) = \nabla_\theta(\int_{L_{\theta^{(k)}}} f(r)\mathrm{d}|r|), \tag{3}$$

where $L_{\theta(k)}$ is the integration path determined by projection configuration $\theta(k)$. We call each path of integration a ray.

With all $\nabla_\theta(\mathcal{R}f^{(k)})(\theta^{(k)})$ calculated and the precondition that the minimum of Eq. (2) is 0, the minimization turns out solving $\Delta\theta$ in a linear equation set $||(\nabla_\theta(\mathcal{R}f^{(k)})(\theta^{(k)})f) \cdot \Delta\theta|| = 0$. Each equation in this set corresponds to a different θ. Noticing the fact that the electron microscope collects all g data with same angular parameters simultaneously, data points with same $(\theta_\alpha, \theta_\beta, \theta_\gamma)$ share the same $\Delta\theta$. With the reduction of variables, the equation set is now over-determined and its least-squares solution is what we are looking for. For every iteration, the reconstruction and corresponding Taylor expansions are recalculated to make sure the error caused by $\Delta\theta$ is always much more significant than error from minimization.

3.3   Time Complexity and Hardware-Based Improvements

According to the algorithm outline, the basic calculation unit of optimization is the solving of operator $\mathcal{R}$, $\nabla_\theta\mathcal{R}$, and $\mathcal{S}$. Compared with naive exhaustive search (NES) method, our method significantly decreases the amount of calculation. The NES method goes through the solution space to find the best configuration match. To eliminate influence by other configuration parameters, each parameter must be searched separately and one $\mathcal{R}$ and one $\mathcal{S}$ operator is carried out during every single trial. Instead, for the sake of gradient descent, our method accomplishes correcting for all configuration parameters in one descent made up with one $\mathcal{R}$ calculation, one $\nabla_\theta(\mathcal{R})$ calculation, and one $\mathcal{S}$. In addition, in order to reduce further, we find that during one descent process, the data usage and calculation structure in calculations of $\mathcal{R}$ and $\nabla_\theta(\mathcal{R})$ have much in common. We also find that during one calculation, one data point in f is used only 1–5 times for multiplication before it's discarded. All these features inspire us to an idea of heterogeneous computing and data reuse. So we firstly input data f and current configuration into an OpenCL kernel. $\mathcal{R}f$ and $\nabla_\theta(\mathcal{R})f$ are then calculated simultaneously to make full use of GPU bandwidth. The rough estimation of theoretical calculation amount is shown in Table 1. In this table, N_p represents the value number of trial for one configuration parameter. Namely, when 3 values in both sides of a given value with fixed interval are tried, N_p is 7. The 4th column in Table 1 shows a specific comparison among methods when $N_p = 7$ and the cost of $\mathcal{R}$ and $\mathcal{S}$ considered to be comparable.

For the reprojection $\mathcal{R}f$ process, which is the most expensive, we make use of Vivado High Level Synthesis (HLS) for acceleration. This tool enables accelerating Clang-base design and exporting RTL as a Vivado's IP core. To adapt for

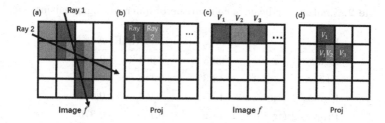

Fig. 2. (a) Ray-based: ray track in data f. (b) Ray-based: data output in data $\mathcal{R}f$. (c) Voxel-based: sequential data read from f. (d) Voxel-based: data output in data $\mathcal{R}f$.

hardware features of FPGA, we rearrange data flow of reprojection process from ray-based to voxel-based to ensure data independency of inner loop. As shown in Fig. 2(a) and (b), ray-based orienting calculate the path of rays in f and load corresponding data. The loaded data is process and then output in $\mathcal{R}f$ accordingly. However The load sections of different rays overlap a lot, which causes huge load conflicts. Those conflicts are unpredictable and make initial interval (II) unbearable. To solve this problem, we read voxel data from f sequentially and find out the rays that contain voxel data as Fig. 2(c) and (d) shows. We find that adjacent voxels always belong to adjacent rays. So we cache the output data instead of saving it until the current voxel is irrelevant to it. In this way pipeline among voxels and be carried out and the II could be reduced.

Table 1. Time complexity comparison. The value 1.4 at row.4 & col.2 is an experimental result of data reuse. The value 5 at row.2 & col.3 is the size of tuple that describe a projection.

Method	Trial cost	Trial per iter.	Specific case
NES	$1 \times \mathcal{R} + 1 \times \mathcal{S}$	$N_p \times 5$	$70 \times \mathcal{R}$
Proposed (w/o data reuse)	$6 \times \mathcal{R} + 1 \times \mathcal{S}$	1	$7 \times \mathcal{R}$
Proposed (w/ data reuse)	$1.4 \times \mathcal{R} + 1 \times \mathcal{S}$	1	$2.4 \times \mathcal{R}$

4   Experiments and Result

The dataset we use for experiment is a conical-tilt projection series collected by FEI Tecnai 12 and 2048×2048 CCD Gatan camera. The sample were tilt to $55°$ and then rotated by $5°$ interval (72 projections in total). One of its projection is displayed in Fig. 3(a). And the test is carried out on a linux platform with $2 \times$E5-2650 v3, 64 GB Memory and Tesla K80. The synthesis tool is Vivado 2019.1 and synthesis configuration is based on Xilinx ZCU102.

Using this dataset as input, we run both proposed method and NES method for alignment. Popular feature-based method [3] does not provide a solution for conical tilt datasets, so it is temporarily excluded. For NES method, we collect the total time cost and the final alignment result. For proposed method,

Table 2. Similarity indicators comparison of different alignment methods.

Method	Avg MSE	Avg RAE	Avg NCC
Raw	92.8	0.991	0.449
NES	18.3	0.188	0.873
Proposed (one iter)	18.3	0.191	0.871
Proposed (two iters)	18.2	0.189	0.870

alignment results and detailed time costs after every iteration are recorded. For every alignment result, we reproject corresponding reconstruction image using configuration determined by the result to obtain reprojection images. Then the similarity between reprojection images and input conical-tilt dataset is evaluated using indicators like mean squared error (MSE), relative average error (RAE), and normalized cross correlation (NCC). The similarity indicators reveal the accuracy of the alignment. Specially, When accuracy is higher, the MSE value is lower, RAE value is lower and NCC value is higher. Table 2 shows the average indicators value of different projections. The projection process, which is the bottleneck, is C-synthesised on Vivado HLS with target ap_clk = 10ns and resource limited by Xilinx ZCU102.

Table 3. Time cost details of methods.

Method	OpenCL init (s)	Reproj (s)	Recon (s)	IO (s)	Total (s)
NES	–	–	–	–	5520
Prop (one iter)	4.5	56.2	50.6	67.0	178.3
Prop (two iters)	9.0	112.4	75.9	134.0	331.3
HLS (reproj only)	II $= 1$	Latency $= 10.6E8$			$\sim$9.2

Except for quantitative evaluation, for visual observation, cross section of reconstruction results by proposed method and NES method is shown in Fig. 3(b) and (c). The sharpness and clarity of images by both methods is comparable.

The time cost information of methods is listed in Table 3. The result shows a significant speed-up of 16.7$\times$ between NES method and proposed method. The HLS simulation for reprojection process also has a 6.6$\times$ speed-up over our well-optimized OpenCL program on Tesla K80.

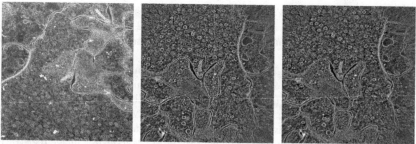

(a) One of the projections (b) Cross section of the re- (c) Cross section of the re-
from experiment dataset   con by prop method after   con by NES method
                            2 iters

Fig. 3. Experimental data and reconstruction results comparison of different alignment methods.

5 Conclusion

Effective alignment for nanometer-scale electron is currently a challenge. Using the gradient-based approach, we have derived a descent method which decomposes the problem into a computational friendly optimization problem. This method is capable of accurate alignment for datasets with no fiducial markers. The experiment results show the reliability and efficiency. Compared with the NES method, our method manage to achieve comparable accuracy with 16.7× efficiency, which enables operators or researchers to get fine reconstruction of ROI almost instantly after data collection. For reprojection related process in our method, a preliminary design based on Xilinx ZCU102 shows a 6.6× acceleration compared with a well-optimized OpenCL program on GPU.

References

1. Fernandez, J.J.: Computational methods for electron tomography. Micron **43**(10), 1010–1030 (2012)
2. Guckenberger, R.: Determination of a common origin in the micrographs of tilt series in three-dimensional electron microscopy. Ultramicroscopy **9**(1–2), 167–173 (1982)
3. Han, R., Bao, Z., Zeng, X., et al.: A joint method for marker-free alignment of tilt series in electron tomography. Bioinformatics **35**(14), i249–i259 (2019)
4. Herman, G.T.: Fundamentals of Computerized Tomography: Image Reconstruction from Projections, pp. 64–68. Springer, London (2009). https://doi.org/10.1007/978-1-84628-723-7
5. Houben, L., Sadan, M.B.: Refinement procedure for the image alignment in high-resolution electron tomography. Ultramicroscopy **111**(9–10), 1512–1520 (2011)
6. Leis, A., Rockel, B., Andrees, L., et al.: Visualizing cells at the nanoscale. Trends Biochem. Sci. **34**(2), 60–70 (2009)
7. Lucas, B.D., Kanade, T.: An iterative image registration technique with an application to stereo vision (1981)

8. Mastronarde, D.N., Held, S.R.: Automated tilt series alignment and tomographic reconstruction in IMOD. J. Struct. Biol. **197**(2), 102–113 (2017)
9. Natterer, F.: The Mathematics of Computerized Tomography. SIAM, Philadelphia (1986)
10. Tian, Q., Öfverstedt, L.G.,: Unit USSCB. Semi-automatically aligned tilt images in electron tomography. In: 2017 International Conference on Intelligent Informatics and Biomedical Sciences (ICIIBMS), pp. 71–75. IEEE (2017)
11. Trampert, P., Bogachev, S., Marniok, N., et al.: Marker detection in electron tomography: a comparative study. Microsc. Microanal. **21**(6), 1591–1601 (2015)
12. Sorzano, C.O.S., Messaoudi, C., Eibauer, M., et al.: Marker-free image registration of electron tomography tilt-series. BMC Bioinform. **10**(1), 124 (2009)
13. Winkler, H., Taylor, K.A.: Accurate marker-free alignment with simultaneous geometry determination and reconstruction of tilt series in electron tomography. Ultramicroscopy **106**(3), 240–254 (2006)

U-Net Fixed-Point Quantization for Medical Image Segmentation

MohammadHossein AskariHemmat[1]([✉]), Sina Honari[2]([✉]), Lucas Rouhier[3]([✉]),
Christian S. Perone[3]([✉]), Julien Cohen-Adad[3]([✉]), Yvon Savaria[1]([✉]),
and Jean-Pierre David[1]([✉])

[1] Ecole Polytechnique Montreal, Montreal, Canada
{mohammadhossein.askari-hemmat,yvon.savaria,
jean-pierre.david}@polymtl.ca
[2] Mila-University of Montreal, Montreal, Canada
sina.honari@umontreal.ca
[3] NeuroPoly Lab, Institute of Biomedical Engineering,
Polytechnique Montreal, Montreal, Canada
{lucas.rouhier,julien.cohen-adad}@polymtl.ca,
christian.perone@gmail.com

Abstract. Model quantization is leveraged to reduce the memory consumption and the computation time of deep neural networks. This is achieved by representing weights and activations with a lower bit resolution when compared to their high precision floating point counterparts. The suitable level of quantization is directly related to the model performance. Lowering the quantization precision (e.g. 2 bits), reduces the amount of memory required to store model parameters and the amount of logic required to implement computational blocks, which contributes to reducing the power consumption of the entire system. These benefits typically come at the cost of reduced accuracy. The main challenge is to quantize a network as much as possible, while maintaining the performance accuracy. In this work, we present a quantization method for the U-Net architecture, a popular model in medical image segmentation. We then apply our quantization algorithm to three datasets: (1) the Spinal Cord Gray Matter Segmentation (GM), (2) the ISBI challenge for segmentation of neuronal structures in Electron Microscopic (EM), and (3) the public National Institute of Health (NIH) dataset for pancreas segmentation in abdominal CT scans. The reported results demonstrate that with only 4 bits for weights and 6 bits for activations, we obtain 8 fold reduction in memory requirements while loosing only 2.21%, 0.57% and 2.09% dice overlap score for EM, GM and NIH datasets respectively. Our fixed point quantization provides a flexible trade-off between accuracy and memory requirement, which is not provided by previous quantization methods for U-Net (Our code is released at https://github.com/hossein1387/U-Net-Fixed-Point-Quantization-for-Medical-Image-Segmentation).

Electronic supplementary material The online version of this chapter (https://doi.org/10.1007/978-3-030-33642-4_13) contains supplementary material, which is available to authorized users.

Keywords: U-Net · Quantization · Deep learning

1   Introduction

Image segmentation, the task of specifying the class of each pixel in an image, is one of the active research areas in the medical imaging domain. In particular, image segmentation for biomedical imaging allows identifying different tissues, biomedical structures, and organs from images to help medical doctors diagnose diseases. However, manual image segmentation is a laborious task. Deep learning methods have been used to automate the process and alleviate the burden of segmenting images manually.

The rise of Deep Learning has enabled patients to have direct access to personal health analysis [1]. Health monitoring apps on smartphones are now capable of monitoring medical risk factors. Medical health centers and hospitals are equipped with pre-trained models used in medical CADs to analyse MRI images [2]. However, developing a high precision model often comes with various costs, such as a higher computational burden and a large model size. The latter requires many parameters to be stored in floating point precision, which demands high hardware resources to store and process images at test time. In medical domains, images typically have high resolution and can also be volumetric (the data has a depth in addition to width and height). Quantizing the neural networks can reduce the feedforward computation time and most importantly the memory burden at inference. After quantization, a high precision (floating point) model is approximated with a lower bit resolution model. The goal is to leverage the advantages of the quantization techniques while maintaining the accuracy of the full precision floating point models. Quantized models can then be deployed on devices with limited memory such as cell-phones, or facilitate processing higher resolution images or bigger volumes of 3D data with the same memory budget. Developing such methods can reduce the required memory to save model parameters potentially up to 32x in memory footprint. In addition, the amount of hardware resources (the number of logic gates) required to perform low precision computing, is much less than a full precision model [3]. In this paper, we propose a fixed point quantization of U-Net [4], a popular segmentation architecture in the medical imaging domain. We provide comprehensive quantization results on the Spinal Cord Gray Matter Segmentation Challenge [5], the ISBI challenge for segmentation of neuronal structures in electron microscopic stacks [6], and the public National Institute of Health (NIH) dataset for pancreas segmentation in abdominal CT scans [7]. In summary, this work makes the following contributions:

- We report the first fixed point quantization results on the U-Net architecture for the medical image segmentation task and show that the current quantization methods available for U-Net are not efficient for the hardware commonly available in the industry.
- We quantify the impact of quantizing the weights and activations on the performance of the U-Net model on three different medical imaging datasets.

– We report results comparable to a full precision segmentation model by using only 6 bits for activation and 4 bits for weights, effectively reducing the weights size by a factor of 8× and the activation size by a factor of 5×.

2 Related Works

2.1 Image Segmentation

Image segmentation is one of the central problems in medical imaging [8], commonly used to detect regions of interest such as tumors. Deep learning approaches have obtained the state-of-the-art results in medical image segmentation [9,10]. One of the favorite architectures used for image segmentation is U-Net [4] or its equivalent architectures proposed around the same time; ReCombinator Networks [11], SegNet [12], and DeconvNet [13], all proposed to maintain pixel level information that is usually lost due to pooling layers. These models use an encoder-decoder architecture with skip connections, where the information in the encoder path is reintroduced by skip connections in the decoder path. This architecture has proved to be quite successful for many applications that require full image reconstruction while changing the modality of the data, as in the image-to-image translation [14], semantic segmentation [4,12,13] or landmark localization [11,15]. While all the aforementioned models propose the same architecture, for simplicity we refer to them as U-Net models. U-Net type models have been very popular in the medical imaging domain and have been also applied to the 3 dimensional (3D) segmentation task [16]. One problem with U-Net is its high usage of memory due to full image reconstruction. All encoded features are required to be kept in memory and then used while reconstructing the final output. This approach can be quite demanding, especially for high resolution or 3D images. Quantization of weights and activations can reduce the required memory for this model, allowing to process images with a higher resolution or with a bigger 3D volume at test time.

2.2 Quantization for Medical Imaging Segmentation

There are two approaches to quantize a neural network, namely deterministic quantization and stochastic quantization [3]. Although DNN quantization has been thoroughly studied [3,17,18], little effort has been done on developing quantization methods for medical image segmentation. In the following, we review recent works in this field.

Quantization in Fully Convolutional Networks: Quantization has been applied to Fully Convolutional Networks (FCN) in biomedical image segmentation [19]. First, a quantization module was added to the suggestive annotation in FCN. In suggestive annotation, instead of using the original dataset, a representative training dataset was used, which in turn increased the accuracy. Next, FCN segmentations were quantized using Incremental Quantization (INQ). Authors report that suggestive annotation with INQ using 7 bits results in accuracy close to or better than those obtained with a full precision model. In FCN, features of different resolutions are upsampled back to the image resolution and merged together right before the final output predictions. This approach is sub-optimal compared to the U-Net which upsamples features only to one higher resolution, allowing the model to process them before they are passed to higher resolution layers. This gradual resolution increase in reconstruction acts as a conditional computation, where the features of higher resolution are computed using the lower resolution features. As reported in [11], this process of conditional computation results in faster convergence time and increased accuracy in the U-Net type architectures compared to the FCN type architectures. Considering the aforementioned advantages of U-Net, in this paper we pursue the quantization of this model.

U-Net Quantization: In [20], the authors propose the first quantization for U-Net. They introduce (1) a parameterized ternary hyperbolic tangent to be used as the activation function, (2) a ternary convolutional method that calculates matrix multiplication very efficiently in the hamming space. They report 15-fold decrease in the memory requirement as well as 10x speed-up at inference compared to the full precision model. Although this method shows significant performance boost, in Sect. 4 we demonstrate that this is not an efficient method for the currently available CPUs and GPUs.

3 Proposed Quantization

We propose fixed point quantization for U-Net. We start with a full precision (32 bit floating point) model as our baseline. We then use the following fixed point quantization function to quantize the parameters (weights and activation) in the inference path:

$$quantize(x, n) = (round(clamp(x, n) << n)) >> n \qquad (1)$$

where the *round* function projects its input to the nearest integer, $<<$ and $>>$ are shift left and right operators, respectively. In our simulation, shift left and right are implemented by multiplication and division in powers of 2. The *clamp* function is defined as:

$$clamp(x, n) = \begin{cases} 2^n - 1 & \text{when} \quad x \geq 2^n - 1 \\ x & \text{when} \quad 0 < x < 2^n - 1 \\ 0 & \text{when} \quad x \leq 0 \end{cases} \qquad (2)$$

Equation (1) quantizes an input $x \in \mathbb{R}$ to the closest value that can be represented by n bits. To map any given number x to its fixed point value we first split the number into its fractional and integer parts using:

$$x_f = abs(x) - floor(abs(x)), x_i = floor(abs(x)) \qquad (3)$$

and then use the following equation to convert x to its fixed point representation using the specified number of bits for the integer ($ibits$) and fractional ($fbits$) parts:

$$to\_fixed\_point(x, ibits, fbits) = sign(x) * quantize(x_i, ibits)$$
$$+ sign(x) * quantize(x_f, fbits) \quad (4)$$

Equation (4) is a fixed point quantization function that maps a floating point number x to the closest fixed point value with $ibits$ integer and $fbits$ fractional bits. Throughout this paper, we use $Q^p i.f$ notation to denote that we are using a fixed point quantization of parameter p by using i bits to represent the integer part and f bits to represent the fractional part. Based on our experiments, we did not benefit from an incremental quantization (INQ) as explained in [17]. Although this method could work for higher precision models, for instance when using fixed point $Q^w 8.8$ (Quantizing weights with 8-bit integer and 8-bit fractional parts), for extreme quantization as in $Q^w 0.4$, learning from scratch gave us the best accuracy with the shortest learning time. As shown in Figure S1, in the full precision case, the weights of all U-Net layers are in $[-1, 1]$ range, hence the integer part for the weight quantization is not required.

3.1 Training

For numerical stability and to verify the gradients can propagate in training, we demonstrate that our quantization is differentiable. Starting from Eq. (2), the derivative is:

$$\forall x \in \mathbb{R}, \forall n \in \mathbb{Z}^+, \quad \frac{\partial}{\partial x} clamp(x, n) = \begin{cases} 0 & \text{when } x \geq 2^n - 1 \\ 1 & \text{when } 0 < x < 2^n - 1 \\ 0 & \text{when } x \leq 0 \end{cases} \quad (5)$$

which is differentiable except on the thresholds. To make it completely differentiable, a straight-through estimator (STE), introduced in [21], is used. The STE passes gradients over the thresholds and also over the *round* function in Eq. (1).

3.2 Observations on U-Net Quantization

Dropout. Dropout [22] is a regularization technique to prevent over-fitting of DNNs. Although it is used in the original implementation of U-Net, we found that when this technique is applied along with quantization, the accuracy drops a lot. Hence, in our implementation, we removed dropout from all layers. This is due to the fact that quantization acts as a strong regularizer, as reported in [3], hence further regularization with dropout is not required. As shown in Figure S2, for each quantized precision, dropout reduces the accuracy, with the gap being even higher for lower precision quantizations.

Full Precision Layers. It is well accepted to keep the first and the last layers in full precision, when applying quantization [3,23]. However, we found that in the segmentation task, keeping the last layer in full precision has much more impact than keeping the first layer in full precision.

Batch Normalization. Batch normalization is a technique that improves the training speed and accuracy of DNN. We used the Pytorch implementation of batchnorm. In training, we use the quantization block after the batchnorm block in each layer such that the batchnorm is first applied using the floating point calculations and then the quantized value is sent to the next layer (hence not quantizing the batchnorm block during training). However, at inference, Pytorch folds the batchnorm parameters into the weights, effectively including batchnorm parameters in the quantized model as part of the quantized weights.

4 Results and Discussion

We implemented the U-Net model and our fixed-point quantizer in Pytorch. We trained our model over 200 epochs with a batch size of 4. We applied our fixed point quantization along with TernaryNet [20] and Binary [18] quantization on three different datasets: GM [5], EM [6], and NIH [7]. For GM and EM datasets, we used an initial learning rate of $1e-3$, and for NIH we used initial learning rate of 0.0025. For all datasets we used Glorot for weight initialization and cosine annealing scheduler to reduce learning rate in training. Please check our repository for the model and training details[1].

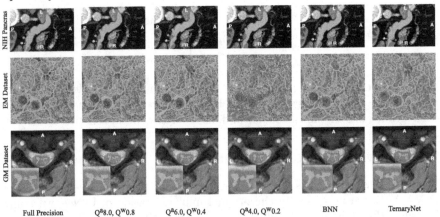

Fig. 1. Sample prediction versus ground truth segmentation results for NIH Pancreas (top), EM (middle) and GM (bottom) datasets. From left to right, the result of different quantization methods and precisions are reported. Segments in ■ show false positive, segments in ■ show false negative and segments in ■ show true positive. (Color figure online)

---

[1] https://github.com/hossein1387/U-Net-Fixed-Point-Quantization-for-Medical-Image-Segmentation.

The NIH pancreas [7] dataset is composed of 82 3D abdominal CT scan and their corresponding pancreas segmentation images. Unfortunately, we did not have access to the pre-processed dataset described in [20], nevertheless, we extracted 512×512 2-D slices from the original dataset and applied a region of interest cropping to get 7059 images of size 176×112. The final dataset contains 7059 176×112 2-D images which are separated into training and testing dataset (respectively 80% and 20%). For GM and EM datasets, we used the provided dataset as described in [5] and [6] respectively. For both EM and GM datasets, we did not used any region of interest cropping and we used images of size 200×200.

The task of image segmentation for GM and NIH pancreas datasets is imbalanced. As suggested in [5], instead of weighted cross-entropy, we used a surrogate loss for the dice similarity coefficient. This loss is referred to as the dice loss and is formulated as $\mathcal{L}_{dice} = \frac{2 \sum_{n=1}^{N} p_n r_n + \epsilon}{\sum_{n=1}^{N} p_n + \sum_{n=1}^{N} r_n + \epsilon}$, where $p_n \in [0, 1]$ and $r_n \in \{0, 1\}$ are prediction and ground truth pixels respectively (with 0 indicating *not-belonging* and 1 indicating *belonging* to the class of interest) and ϵ is the noise added for numerical stability. For the EM dataset, using a weighted sum of cross entropy and dice loss produced the best results.

Figure 1 along with Table 1 show the impact of different quantization methods on the aforementioned datasets. Considering the NIH dataset, Fig. 1(top) and Table 1 show that despite using only 1 and 2 bits to represent network parameters, Binary and TernaryNet quantizations produce results that are close to the full precision model. However, for other datasets, our fixed point $Q^a6.0$, $Q^w0.4$ quantization surpasses Binary and TernaryNet quantization. The other important factor here is how efficient these quantization techniques can be implemented using the current CPUs and GPUs hardware. At the time of writing this paper, there is no commercially available CPU or GPU that can efficiently store and load sub-8-bit parameters of a neural network, which leaves us to use custom functions to do bit manipulation to make sub-8-bit quantization more efficient. Moreover, in the case of TernaryNet, to apply floating point scaling factors after ternary convolutions, floating point operations are required. Our fixed point quantization uses only integer operations, which requires less hardware footprint and use less power compared to floating point operations. Finally, TernaryNet uses Tanh instead of ReLU for the activations. Using hyperbolic tangent as an activation function increases training time [24] and execution time at inference. To verify it, we evaluated the performance of ReLU and Tanh in a simple neural network with 3 fully connected layers. We used the Intel's Open-Vino [25] inference engine together with high performance `gemm_blas` and `avx2` instructions. Table 2 reports the results obtained when ReLU is used instead of Tanh at training and it shows that inference time can decrease by up to 8 times. These results can be extended to U-Net, since activation inference time is a direct function of the input size. To compensate for the computation time, TernaryNet implements an efficient ternary convolution that can decrease processing time by up to 8 times. At inference, an efficient Tanh function that uses only two comparators can be implemented to perform Tanh for ternary values.

Considering accuracy, when Tanh is used as an activation function, the full precision accuracy is lower compared to ReLU [20]. We observe similar behavior in the results reported in Table 1. Our fixed point quantizer provides a flexible trade-off between accuracy and memory, which makes it a practical solution for the current CPUs and GPUs, as it does not require floating-point operations, and leverages the more efficient ReLU function. As opposed to BNN and TernaryNet quantizations, Table 1 shows that our approach for quantization of U-Net provides consistent results over 3 different datasets.

Table 1. Dice scores of the quantized U-Net models on EM (left) GM (middle) and NIH (right) datasets. The last two rows show results for Binary and TernaryNet quantizations. Other rows report results obtained for different weights and activations quantization precisions. For the GM and EM datasets, we also report results when Tanh is used instead of ReLU as the activation function.

Quantization			EM dataset		GM dataset		NIH panceas
Activation	Weight	Parameter size	Dice score ReLU	Dice score Tanh	Dice score ReLU	Dice score Tanh	Dice score
Full Precision		18.48 MBytes	94.05	93.02	56.32	56.26	75.69
Q8.8	Q8.8	9.23 MBytes	92.02	91.08	56.11	56.01	74.61
Q8.0	Q0.8	4.61 MBytes	92.21	88.42	56.10	53.78	73.05
Q6.0	Q0.4	2.31 MBytes	91.03	90.93	55.85	52.34	73.48
Q4.0	Q0.2	1.15 MBytes	79.80	54.23	51.80	48.23	71.77
BNN [18]		0.56 MBytes	78.53	–	31.44	–	72.56
TernaryNet [20]		1.15 MBytes	–	82.66	–	43.02	73.9

Table 2. Comparing ReLU and Tanh run time using Intel's OpenVino [25]. Each row illustrates the execution time for a layer of a neural network in micro seconds. It demonstrates that using Tanh as activation can increase execution time by up to 8 times compared to ReLU.

Layer type	Instruction type	Execution time in μs Tanh	Execution time in μs ReLU	Performance Gain of using ReLU over Tanh	Tensor dimension
Activation	jit_avx2_FP32	30	5	6	[100, 100]
FullyConnected	gemm_blas_FP32	20	19	–	–
FullyConnected	gemm_blas_FP32	860	527	–	–
Activation	jit_avx2_FP32	77	9	8.6	[100, 300]

5   Conclusion

In this work, we proposed a fixed point quantization method for the U-Net architecture and evaluated it on the medical image segmentation task. We reported quantization results on three different segmentation datasets and showed that our fixed point quantization produces more accurate and also more consistent results over all these datasets compared to other quantization techniques. We also demonstrated that Tanh, as the activation function, reduces the base-line accuracy and also adds a computational complexity in both training and inference. Our proposed fixed-point quantization technique provides a trade-off between accuracy and the required memory. It does not require floating-point computation and it is more suitable for the currently available CPUs and GPUs hardware.

References

1. Miotto, R., et al.: Deep learning for healthcare: review, opportunities and challenges. Brief. Bioinform. **19**, 1236–1246 (2017)
2. Thaler, S., Menkovski, V.: The role of deep learning in improving healthcare. Data Science for Healthcare, pp. 75–116. Springer, Cham (2019). https://doi.org/10.1007/978-3-030-05249-2_3
3. Hubara, I., et al.: Quantized neural networks: training neural networks with low precision weights and activations. JMLR **18**, 6869–6898 (2018)
4. Ronneberger, O., Fischer, P., Brox, T.: U-Net: convolutional networks for biomedical image segmentation. In: Navab, N., Hornegger, J., Wells, W.M., Frangi, A.F. (eds.) MICCAI 2015. LNCS, vol. 9351, pp. 234–241. Springer, Cham (2015). https://doi.org/10.1007/978-3-319-24574-4_28
5. Prados, F., et al.: Spinal cord grey matter segmentation challenge. NeuroImage **152**, 312–329 (2017)
6. Cardona, A., et al.: An integrated micro-and macroarchitectural analysis of the drosophila brain by computer-assisted serial section electron microscopy. PLoS Biol. **8**, e1000502 (2010)
7. Roth, H.R., et al.: DeepOrgan: multi-level deep convolutional networks for automated pancreas segmentation. In: Navab, N., Hornegger, J., Wells, W.M., Frangi, A.F. (eds.) MICCAI 2015. LNCS, vol. 9349, pp. 556–564. Springer, Cham (2015). https://doi.org/10.1007/978-3-319-24553-9_68
8. Pham, D.L., et al.: Current methods in medical image segmentation. Annu. Rev. Biomed. Eng. **2**, 315–337 (2000)
9. Litjens, G., et al.: A survey on deep learning in medical image analysis. Med. Image Anal. **42**, 60–88 (2017)
10. Shen, D., et al.: Deep learning in medical image analysis. Annu. Rev. Biomed. Eng. **19**, 221–248 (2017)
11. Honari, S., et al.: Recombinator networks: learning coarse-to-fine feature aggregation. In: CVPR (2016)
12. Badrinarayanan, V., et al.: SegNet: a deep convolutional encoder-decoder architecture for image segmentation. TPAMI **39**, 2481–2495 (2017)
13. Noh, H., et al.: Learning deconvolution network for semantic segmentation. In: ICCV (2015)
14. Isola, P., et al.: Image-to-image translation with conditional adversarial networks. In: CVPR (2017)

15. Newell, A., Yang, K., Deng, J.: Stacked hourglass networks for human pose estimation. In: Leibe, B., Matas, J., Sebe, N., Welling, M. (eds.) ECCV 2016. LNCS, vol. 9912, pp. 483–499. Springer, Cham (2016). https://doi.org/10.1007/978-3-319-46484-8_29

16. Çiçek, Ö., Abdulkadir, A., Lienkamp, S.S., Brox, T., Ronneberger, O.: 3D U-Net: learning dense volumetric segmentation from sparse annotation. In: Ourselin, S., Joskowicz, L., Sabuncu, M.R., Unal, G., Wells, W. (eds.) MICCAI 2016. LNCS, vol. 9901, pp. 424–432. Springer, Cham (2016). https://doi.org/10.1007/978-3-319-46723-8_49

17. Zhou, A., et al.: Incremental network quantization: Towards lossless CNNs with low-precision weights. CoRR (2017)

18. Courbariaux, M., et al.: BinaryConnect: training deep neural networks with binary weights during propagations. In: NeurIPS (2015)

19. Xu, X., et al.: Quantization of fully convolutional networks for accurate biomedical image segmentation. In: CVPR (2018)

20. Heinrich, M.P., et al.: TernaryNet: Faster deep model inference without GPUs for medical 3D segmentation using sparse and binary convolutions. CoRR (2018)

21. Hinton, G., et al.: Neural networks for machine learning, video lectures. Coursera (2012)

22. Srivastava, N., et al.: Dropout: a simple way to prevent neural networks from overfitting. JMLR **15**, 1929–1958 (2014)

23. Tang, W., et al.: How to train a compact binary neural network with high accuracy? In: AAAI (2017)

24. Krizhevsky, A., et al.: ImageNet classification with deep convolutional neural networks. In: Advances in Neural Information Processing Systems, vol. 25. Curran Associates, Inc. (2012)

25. Deuermeyer, D., Andrey, Z., Amy, R., Fritz, B.: Release notes for intel® distribution of openvino™ toolkit (2019). Accessed 13 June 2019

Second International Challenge on Correction of Brainshift with Intra-Operative Ultrasound (CuRIOUS 2019)

Registration of Ultrasound Volumes Based on Euclidean Distance Transform

Luca Canalini[1,2(✉)], Jan Klein[1], Dorothea Miller[3], and Ron Kikinis[1,2,4]

[1] Fraunhofer MEVIS, Institute for Digital Medicine, Bremen, Germany
luca.canalini@mevis.fraunhofer.de
[2] Medical Imaging Computing, University of Bremen, Bremen, Germany
[3] Department of Neurosurgery, University Hospital Knappschaftskrankenhaus, Bochum, Germany
[4] Surgical Planning Laboratory, Brigham and Women's Hospital, Harvard Medical School, Boston, USA

Abstract. During neurosurgical operations, surgeons can decide to acquire intraoperative data to better proceed with the removal of a tumor. A valid option is given by ultrasound (US) imaging, which can be easily obtained at subsequent surgical stages, giving therefore multiple updates of the resection cavity. To improve the efficacy of the intraoperative guidance, neurosurgeons may benefit from having a direct correspondence between anatomical structures identified at different US acquisitions. In this context, the commonly available neuronavigation systems already provide registration methods, which however are not enough accurate to overcome the anatomical changes happening during resection. Therefore, our aim with this work is to improve the registration of intraoperative US volumes. In the proposed methodology, first a distance mapping of automatically segmented anatomical structures is computed and then the transformed images are utilized in the registration step. Our solution is tested on a public dataset of 17 cases, where the average landmark registration error between volumes acquired at the beginning and at the end of neurosurgical procedures is reduced from 3.55 mm to 1.27 mm.

Keywords: Ultrasound · Registration · Distance transform

1 Introduction

Before starting a neurosurgical procedure for tumor removal, preoperative data is usually acquired to better plan the successive resection. The most common option is given by magnetic resonance imaging, which can also be accessed during the ongoing surgical procedure to have a better understanding of the resection. In fact, neuronavigation systems can be used to link an intracranial pin-pointed location to the corresponding position in the preoperative data. However, the resection of the tumor and the related anatomical modifications in the surrounding tissues alter the initial configuration of the brain. As consequence,

© Springer Nature Switzerland AG 2019
L. Zhou et al. (Eds.): LABELS 2019/HAL-MICCAI 2019/CuRIOUS 2019, LNCS 11851, pp. 127–135, 2019.
https://doi.org/10.1007/978-3-030-33642-4_14

the anatomical structures will be in another conformation with respect to the one observed in the preplanning data [1], which soon becomes unreliable during neurosurgery. To obtain an updated view of the resection cavity, neurosurgeons can collect intraoperative US data during the resection itself [2,3]. These images can be acquired at different stages of the procedure, for example at the beginning of the surgery, just before opening the dura mater, in order to have an initial estimation of which tissues have to be removed. Moreover, a further acquisition can be done at the end of the resection, to detect possible tumor residual. However, the quality of US images decreases in subsequent acquisitions [4]. Thus, for a better comprehension of the US data obtained at the end of the resection, it would be useful to establish a direct mapping between these images and those acquired at the beginning of the surgery, which have a higher quality. A common solution is provided by neuronavigation systems, which can track the US probe locations and compute a registration between the different acquisitions. However, the generally available systems provide a registration solution which is not enough accurate to model the anatomical deformations happening at subsequent stages. Thus, we propose here an automatic method to improve the registration of US volumes acquired at the beginning and at the end of the surgical operation.

In the context of US-US registration for neurosurgical procedures, some solutions have been already proposed to align volumes acquired before and after resection. For example, the authors in [5] utilized an intensity-based registration method to improve the visualization of volumetric US images. The authors in [6] developed a non-rigid registration approach, in which they proposed a methodology to discard non-corresponding regions between subsequent US acquisitions. The same method has been used in [7]. In another solution [8], the authors aimed to improve the previous algorithm by introducing a symmetric deformation field and an efficient second-order minimization for a better convergence of the method. Then, another method to register pre- and post-resection US volumes was proposed by [9], in which the authors presented a landmark-based registration method. More recently, we provided a segmentation-based method to register US volumes: corresponding structures in US volumes are segmented and then used to guide the registration task [10].

We introduce here a solution which in the first step utilizes the segmentation results obtained in our previous work. Furthermore, it subsequently applies a Euclidean distance operator on automatically segmented anatomical structures and then uses the transformed masks to guide the registration task.

2   Method

Our experiments are conducted by using MeVisLab, on a computer equipped with an Intel Core i7 and a GeForce GTX 1080 (8 GB).

2.1   Euclidean Distance Transform

The first step of our method includes the generation of a distance mapping of automatically segmented brain structures. Regarding the segmentation step, the same methodology has been proposed in our previous solution [10], where a more detailed description is also available. The anatomical elements utilized in our method are the main sulci and falx cerebri. In fact, they clearly appear in US acquisitions due to their *hyperechogenicity* and, moreover, remain visible in subsequent stages, representing valid elements to guide the registration task. To perform the segmentation step, we utilized a convolutional neural network (CNN) model based on the 3D U-Net [11]. With respect to the original architecture, the original depth is reduced to two levels, and a dropout with a value of 0.4 is introduced in order to prevent the network from overfitting. For training, we manually segment the main hyperechogenic structures of interest in 17 US volumes acquired before resection from [12]. A patch size of (30,30,30), padding of (8,8,8) and a batch size of 15 samples have been utilized, and the learning rate has been set to 0.001. The best-trained model was saved according to the highest Jaccard index reached during training and then it was used to segment anatomical structures in volumes acquired in the before- and after-resection stages [12].

Differently from our previous work, a distance mapping is then applied to the automatically generated masks. Regarding this, we can think of a binary image as composed of two different classes, pixels with 0-value in the background (Bg) and pixels with 1-value in the foreground (Fg)

$$I(x, y, z) = \{Fg, Bg\} \tag{1}$$

The distance of each pixel of the foreground from the nearest pixel of the background can be computed. The distance mapping $I_d(x, y, z)$ of the whole image can be expressed as

$$I_d = \begin{cases} 0 & I(x, y, z) \in \{Bg\} \\ min(||x - x_0, y - y_0, z - z_0||, \forall I(x_0, y_0, z_0) \in Bg) & I(x, y, z) \in \{Fg\} \end{cases} \tag{2}$$

Different distance metrics $||x, y, z||$ can be used to compute the transformation, and one of the most common is the Euclidean distance which computes the L2 norm

$$||x, y, z|| = \sqrt{x^2 + y^2 + z^2} \tag{3}$$

In the proposed methodology, we applied the Euclidean distance transform on the automatically generated masks.

2.2 Registration

The transformed masks are utilized to guide the registration task, which has been modified with respect to our previous solution. The proposed method is a variational image registration approach based on [13], in which the correct registration of two volumes corresponds to the global minimum of a discretized objective function. This function is composed of a distance measure, defining the similarity between the deformed template image and the reference image, and a regularizer, limiting the range of possible transformations in the deformable step. In the proposed solution, we respectively chose the normalized gradient field distance (NGF) measure and the curvature regularizer. Moreover, the choice of the optimal transformation parameters has been conducted by using the quasi-Newton l-BGFS [14], due to its speed and memory efficiency. For the registration of the US volumes acquired before and after resection, a solution able to compensate the complex anatomical modifications happening in the resection should be proposed. Thus, our methodology includes an initial parametric step, followed by a non-parametric one. First, the parametric approach utilizes the information provided by the optical tracking systems as an initial guess and then a rigid transformation is performed. In this stage, to speed the optimization process, the images are registered at a resolution one-level coarser compared to the original one. Secondly, the transformation obtained during the parametric registration is used to initialize the non-parametric step. In this stage, to reduce the chance to reach a local minimum, a multilevel technique is introduced: the images are sequentially registered at three different scales. As output of the registration step, the deformed template image is provided.

3   Evaluation

Our method is tested on 17 cases of the RESECT dataset [12]. Each case includes two volumes, the first one acquired after craniotomy but before opening the dura mater, the second one at the end of the resection. The corresponding surgical procedures include only resections of low-grade gliomas (tumor of grade II) in adult patients. Corresponding anatomical landmarks are acquired among the two stages and an initial target registration error (TRE) is provided for each patient, together with a mean target registration error (mTRE) and the corresponding standard deviation (sd). In our methodology, the template and reference entries are respectively the volumes acquired before and after resection. The generated deformation field is directly applied to the landmarks acquired after removal, which are therefore registered to the corresponding ones in the pre-section stage. Regarding the chosen hyperechogenic structures, the first two images of Fig. 1 show the same sulcus segmented in the volumes acquired before and after resection (Fig. 1a and b). In Fig. 1c a 3D section of the same structure visualized in Fig. 1b is provided. Regarding the registration step, TREs computed before and after applying our registration are available in Table 1. By taking as example the same structure of Fig. 1, Fig. 2b shows the registered landmarks in comparison to the original disposition in Fig. 2a. Moreover, in Fig. 3 the first row displays a section of the volume obtained after resection. Furthermore, Fig. 3a displays the initial displacement between the segmented structure in the pre- and post-resection stages. On the contrary, Fig. 3b shows a better overlay between the segmented elements registered with our methodology. In the second row, a section of the same structures is visualized in 3D. Yellow arrows in Fig. 3c indicate the correct direction in which the template image should move (Fig. 3d). The last row of Fig. 3 shows the overlay of the two volumes before and after registration. The whole procedure, including all steps previously described, takes a mean of 38.34 s per each volume.

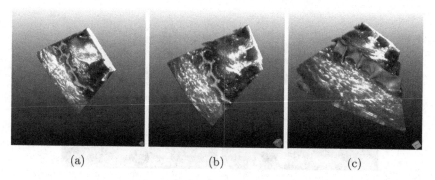

(a)   (b)   (c)

Fig. 1. The same sulcus segmented in corresponding volumes acquired before and after resection stages (Fig. 1a and b). Figure 1c shows a partial view of the 3D segmentation of the same structure of Fig. 1b

Table 1. Registration results in millimeter.

Volume	Landmarks	Before registration	After registration
1	13	5.80 (3.62–7.22)	1.05 (0.28–2.48)
2	10	3.65 (1.71–6.72)	2.32 (0.42–4.16)
3	11	2.91 (1.53–4.30)	1.39 (0.55–2.24)
4	12	2.22 (1.25–2.94)	0.81 (0.25–1.80)
6	11	2.12 (0.75–3.82)	1.62 (0.39–4.65)
7	18	3.62 (1.19–5.93)	1.25 (0.25–3.15)
12	11	3.97 (2.58–6.35)	0.87 (0.20–1.82)
14	17	0.63 (0.17–1.76)	0.62 (0.32–1.10)
15	15	1.63 (0.62–2.69)	0.80 (0.27–1.81)
16	17	3.13 (0.82–5.41)	1.26 (0.22–3.91)
17	11	5.71 (4.25–8.03)	1.51 (0.47–5.59)
18	13	5.29 (2.94–9.26)	1.53 (0.30–3.61))
19	13	2.05 (0.43–3.24)	1.60 (0.39–3.45))
21	9	3.35 (2.34–5.64)	1.82 (0.25–5.12)
24	14	2.61 (1.96–3.41)	0.90 (0.24–2.33)
25	12	7.61 (6.40–10.25)	1.00 (0.30–2.44)
27	12	3.98 (3.09–4.82)	1.24 (0.35–2.74))
Mean ± sd	12.9 ± 2.6	3.55 ± 1.76	1.27 ± 0.44

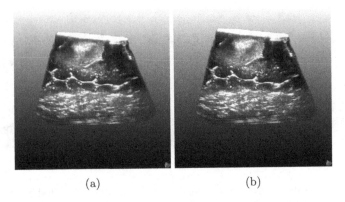

(a)   (b)

Fig. 2. Registration results for landmarks. In both images, a 3D section of the volume acquired before resection is provided, with a subset of related landmarks (green). The positions of the landmarks acquired after resection (purple) are provided before and after registration. (Color figure online)

4 Discussion

The hyperechogenic structures of interest are correctly identified in both stages, as shown for the segmented sulcus in Fig. 1. Moreover, the chosen structures are useful elements to guide the further registration step. In fact, Table 1 shows that the initial mTRE is reduced from 3.55 mm to 1.27 mm and the TRE of each case decreases. For the dataset of interest, the proposed method gives proof to correctly register US volumes acquired before and after resection. Visual results related to the registration of the structures of interest in Fig. 3 confirm the numerical findings. Moreover, when the deformation field is applied to the landmarks (Fig. 2), we can notice how the updated position of the landmarks acquired after resection is closer to the corresponding landmarks acquired in the volume before resection.

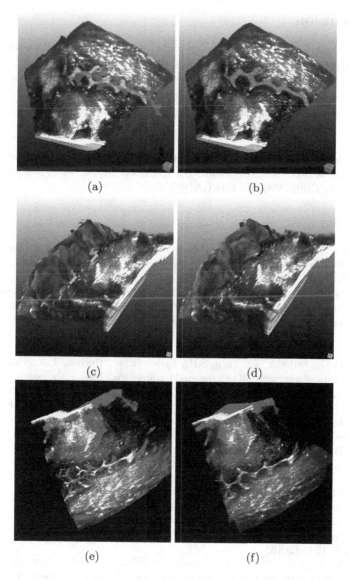

Fig. 3. Registration results for the same sulcus segmented in the before resection (purple) and in the after resection (green) stages. In the first row, a section of the volume acquired after section is displayed, together with 2D views of the segmented structure from both stages. Figure 3a shows how extended is the original displacement of the masks before registration, which is reduced after applying the proposed method (Fig. 3b. In the second row, the same evidence is provided with 3D visualization of the same structure. Then, in the last row an overlay of the original volumes before (Fig. 3e) and after (Fig. 3f) registration is shown. (Color figure online)

5 Conclusion

Our method performs well on the volumes of the RESECT dataset acquired before and after resection. The proposed solution improves the registration results with respect to our previous work [10], which however has been tested on a larger number of cases. Therefore, to better verify the efficacy of the solution, as future work we could decide to apply the proposed solution on a larger set of data.

Acknowledgements. This work was funded by the H2020 Marie-Curie ITN TRA-BIT (765148) project. Moreover, Prof. Dr. Kikinis is supported by NIH grants P41 EB015902, P41 EB015898, and U24 CA180918.

References

1. Gerard, I.J., Kersten-Oertel, M., Petrecca, K., Sirhan, D., Hall, J.A., Collins, D.L.: Brain shift in neuronavigation of brain tumors: a review. Med. Image Anal. **35**, 403–420 (2017)
2. Unsgaard, G., Ommedal, S., Muller, T., Gronningsaeter, A., Nagelhus Hernes, T.A.: Neuronavigation by intraoperative three-dimensional ultrasound: initial experience during brain tumor resection. Neurosurgery **50**(4), 804–812 (2002)
3. Unsgaard, G., et al.: Intra-operative 3D ultrasound in neurosurgery. Acta Neurochir. **148**(3), 235–253 (2006)
4. Rygh, O.M., Selbekk, T., Torp, S.H., Lydersen, S., Hernes, T.A., Unsgaard, G.: Comparison of navigated 3D ultrasound findings with histopathology in subsequent phases of glioblastoma resection. Acta Neurochir. **150**, 1033–1042 (2008)
5. Mercier, L., Araujo, D., Haegelen, C., Del Maestro, R.F., Petrecca, K., Collins, D.L.: Registering pre- and postresection 3-dimensional ultrasound for improved visualization of residual brain tumor. Ultrasound Med. Biol. **39**(1), 16–29 (2013)
6. Rivaz, H., Collins, D.L.: Near real-time robust nonrigid registration of volumetric ultrasound images for neurosurgery. Ultrasound Med. Biol. **41**(2), 574–587 (2015)
7. Rivaz, H., Collins, D.L.: Deformable registration of preoperative MR, pre-resection ultrasound, and post-resection ultrasound images of neurosurgery. Int. J. Comput. Assist. Radiol. Surg. **10**(7), 1017–1028 (2015)
8. Hang, Z., Rivaz, H.: Registration of pre- and postresection ultrasound volumes with noncorresponding regions in neurosurgery. IEEE J. Biomed. Health Inform. **20**, 1240–1249 (2016)
9. Machado, I., et al.: Non-rigid registration of 3D ultrasound for neurosurgery using automatic feature detection and matching. Int. J. Comput. Assist. Radiol. Surg. **13**(10), 1525–1538 (2018)
10. Canalini, L., Klein, J., Miller, D., Kikinis, R.: Segmentation-based registration of ultrasound volumes for glioma resection in image-guided neurosurgery. Int. J. Comput. Assist. Radiol. Surg. **14**(10), 1697–1713 (2019)
11. Çiçek, Ö., Abdulkadir, A., Lienkamp, S.S., Brox, T., Ronneberger, O.: 3D U-Net: Learning Dense Volumetric Segmentation from Sparse Annotation. CoRR, 1606.06650 (2016)
12. Xiao, Y., Fortin, M., Unsgård, G., Rivaz, H., Reinertsen, I.: REtroSpective Evaluation of Cerebral Tumors (RESECT): a clinical database of pre-operative MRI and intra-operative ultrasound in low-grade glioma surgeries. Med. Phys. **44**(7), 3875–3882 (2017)

13. Modersitzki, J.: Flexible algorithms for image registration. SIAM (2009)
14. Liu, D.C., Nocedal, J.: On the limited memory BFGS method for large scale optimization. Math. Program. **45**(1–3), 503–528 (1989)

Landmark-Based Evaluation of a Block-Matching Registration Framework on the RESECT Pre- and Intra-operative Brain Image Data Set

David Drobny[1,3]($\boxtimes$)(iD), Marta Ranzini[2,3](iD), Sébastien Ourselin[3](iD),
Tom Vercauteren[3](iD), and Marc Modat[3](iD)

[1] Wellcome/EPSRC Centre for Interventional and Surgical Sciences, University College London, London WC1E 6BT, UK
d.drobny.17@ucl.ac.uk
[2] Medical Physics and Biomedical Engineering Department, University College London, London WC1E 6BT, UK
marta.ranzini.15@ucl.ac.uk
[3] School of Biomedical Engineering & Imaging Sciences, King's College London, King's Health Partners, St Thomas' Hospital, London SE1 7EH, UK
{sebastien.ourselin,tom.vercauteren,marc.modat}@kcl.ac.uk

Abstract. In this paper, we describe the application of an established block-matching based registration method to the CuRIOUS 2019 MICCAI registration challenge. Directional and symmetric approaches with different parameters are evaluated to select the most suitable setting of this fully automatic and general registration method. The results can be used as a baseline, for example when evaluating methods specialised in ultrasound (US) to MRI registration or registration of different interventional US (iUS) data. This work is a continuation of our contribution to the CuRIOUS 2018 challenge. We provide a more extensive analysis of main parameters as well as add pre- to post-resection iUS registration to the previous MRI-iUS registration. The proposed approach achieves an average target registration error of 2.68 mm and 1.92 mm for the MR-iUS and the iUS-iUS task respectively.

Keywords: Block-matching · Symmetric registration · Resection · Brain shift · Fully automatic · MRI · iUS

1 Introduction

Brain tumour resection procedures can benefit from navigated surgery systems which allow displaying tumour segmentations, surgery plans, or regions of interest. The accuracy of the displayed information can be impaired by changes in the soft brain tissue. Intra-operative imaging techniques such as interventional ultrasound (iUS) can provide data of the current anatomy which can be used

L. Zhou et al. (Eds.): LABELS 2019/HAL-MICCAI 2019/CuRIOUS 2019, LNCS 11851, pp. 136–144, 2019.
https://doi.org/10.1007/978-3-030-33642-4_15

to update pre-operative images. However accurate image registration is required to establish meaningful correspondences of the pre- and intra-operative images. The CuRIOUS 2019 MICCAI challenge aims at comparing state of the art registration methods in two tasks: aligning pre-operative MR images with iUS images before tumour resection (in continuation of the 2018 challenge [7]) and aligning iUS images before and after resection.

In this work, we evaluate a method which uses a block-matching approach to fully automatically solve both registration tasks. This registration method is well established and yields good results in different applications [2,3]. As this approach is not specialised to the registration challenge at hand, the results can provide a baseline when comparing to domain-specific approaches. We provide an analysis of important parameters of the registration framework and insight into its limitations. We finally demonstrate registration results for this data set that can be achieved by an out of the box approach.

2   Methods

Registration algorithms that align one image to a fixed reference image can introduce a directional bias, i.e. results and derived metrics can vary depending on which image is kept fixed and which is transformed. This has been shown, for example, in brain atrophy evaluation [9]. Symmetric approaches overcome this bias by generating a transformation that can be applied in both directions. Other desirable properties like improved capture range, higher accuracy and robustness of the symmetric approach were shown in [4]. The registration framework used for this application is published as part of the NiftyReg open-source software package (version 1.5.61) [5].

2.1   Block-Matching Based Registration

In the block-matching algorithm, first a set of correspondences of reference image and warped floating image blocks are established independently and then simultaneously used to determine the global transformation parameters by least trimmed squares (LTS) regression [6]. The blocks are determined by splitting the floating image into uniform blocks of four voxel edge length (default value). To improve robustness, only a percentage v of blocks with the highest variance of intensity values is kept in this step. Each of those blocks is compared to all reference image blocks that overlap with at least one voxel. The block with the highest absolute normalised cross-correlation (NCC) is selected as correspondence. The block matching approach is embedded in a multi-resolution scheme with ln levels. The registration is first computed on the $(ln-1)$-times down-sampled image. These results are used as an initialisation of the next finer resolution level. This procedure is repeated until the full resolution images are registered. The coarse-to-fine approach helps to avoid local minima and increases the capture range of the registration while enabling a speed-up of the computation.

2.2 Symmetric Registration

Symmetric registration approaches avoid the need to choose which image to select as reference and floating image. Also, it avoids bias, introduced by non-symmetric methods otherwise. Performing both directions of registration at each iteration allows the resulting transformations to be averaged in log-space [4]. This averaged transformation can be used in one direction and its inverse in the opposite direction and can thus be considered bias-free.

2.3 Experimental Set-Up

The dataset used for this work was published as the RESECT database [8]. It contains 23 cases with pre-operative T2 FLAIR and T1-weighted MR images as well as intra-operative ultrasounds images at three time points of the procedure: after craniotomy and before opening the dura, during the tumour resection, and after resection. Each case is provided with landmark pairs, indicating the correspondence of anatomical landmarks in certain image pairs. Based on those landmarks, the mean target registration error (mTRE) provides a useful metric to describe the quality of the registration result.

In the context of the CuRIOUS 2018 challenge, we showed that the FLAIR MR images are more suitable for the multi-modal registration task compared to the T1-weighted MR images [1]. Accordingly, the experiments of this work focus on the FLAIR MR images as well. The possibility of combining information of both MR images is not being investigated, as the registration framework works on image pairs only. This year's challenge extends the pre-operative MR to intra-operative US registration task by before and after resection iUS image registration. For both tasks of the challenge, the following three registration settings are investigated: either image used as reference image and the symmetric approach. For each setting, both rigid and affine transformations are evaluated. Furthermore, two important parameters of the registration algorithm—the number of levels of the pyramidal approach, ln, and the percentage of matched blocks, v—are varied. The values used for ln are $2, 3$, and 4 and the values for v are $10, 25$, and 100. All other parameters are kept as the default values. This totals in 54 configurations per registration task. Based on thresholding each US image with the background value, a mask is generated. Dilating this mask of the iUS image before resection by 20 mm provides an estimate of the search space in the MR image and is used as the MR image mask. The MR image is also cropped to the bounding box of the mask to reduce the image size. No further pre-processing or resampling of the image volumes was applied. The initial alignment of the images was derived from the image header information which was generated by tracking the US probe.

3 Results

The comparison of various registration settings for MR-iUS alignment is shown in Fig. 1. This shows that the choice of reference image has a significant impact on accuracy. Using the MR image as reference leads to much larger mean target registration errors (mTREs) than the iUS image. The symmetric approach, which combines the two directed registrations, yields results close to the better directional one although almost always worse. The best results have a trimmed mean (i.e. ignoring outliers) around 2 mm while the worst result goes up to 60 mm.

In the comparison of the rigid and affine results of each experiment, the rigid transformation outperforms the affine approach in most cases. Only in the setting with the iUS image taken as reference and combined with low values of ln does the affine transformation provide better registration results than the rigid approach. Increasing the percentage of matched blocks moderately improves the average mTRE and reduces the standard deviation over all the experiments, at the expense of increased computational load. When increasing the number of pyramidal levels, ln, poor results become worse, especially for the affine registrations. This creates a bigger difference between rigid and affine registration for higher levels of ln, making the rigid ones more consistent.

The mTREs of the iUS-iUS registration task (Fig. 2) show a consistent pattern across all parameter settings of ln and v. Using the iUS image after tumour resection as reference leads to the best results with an average mTRE around 2 mm, while the other direction and the symmetric approach show very similar results around 5 mm to 6 mm. In this registration task, affine transformations increase the mTRE in most cases. Similarly to MR-iUS results, higher values of ln increase the impairment of using the affine transformation. Increasing v shows only negligible effects on the mTRE, except for the experiment with the highest ln: Here the lowest value of v significantly increases the mTRE of the affine registration using the iUS after resection as reference, while higher values of v yield results in the same magnitude of all other parameter settings.

Following the evaluation criteria of the CuRIOUS challenge, we select the setting that provides the lowest average mTRE across all available test subjects. Based on the results at hand, we chose the following parameters for both registration tasks: $v = 25$, $ln = 2$. While, for the multi-modal registration task, the affine transformation model yields better results, for the iUS-iUS task the rigid one is chosen instead. Examples of the registration results are visualised in Fig. 3 and show good alignment of structures in both registration tasks. To generate a reference registration which provides the best possible registration given the evaluation metric of mTRE, we computed the affine transformation that minimises the mean landmark distance. The mean TRE of this transformation is referred to as oracle. For both registration tasks, the mTRE of each test case for the rigid and affine registration with the selected parameters is displayed along with the initial landmark distance and the oracle result in Tables 1 and 2.

The average run time of the affine registration for the MR-iUS registration task is 72 s with GPU utilisation (201 s on CPU only) and 23 s (89 s) for the rigid registration of the iUS-iUS task on a computer with AMD Ryzen Threadripper 1950X CPU and NVIDIA Quadro P6000 GPU.

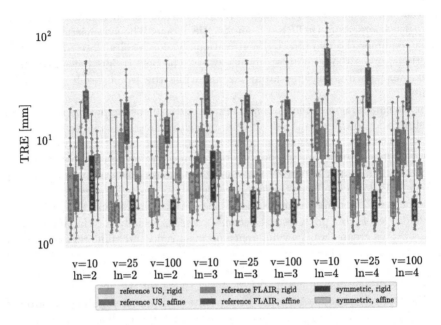

Fig. 1. Boxplots of the mean TREs of all experiments of the MR-iUS registration task. The mTRE of each case is displayed as a dot on top of the boxplot.

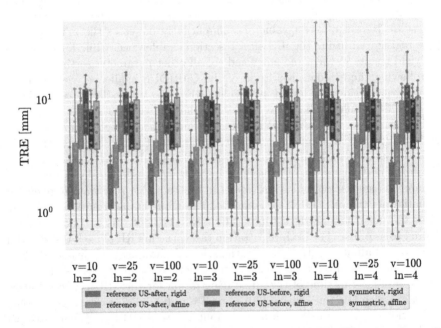

Fig. 2. Boxplots of the mean TREs of all experiments of the iUS-iUS registration task. The mTRE of each case is displayed as a dot on top of the boxplot.

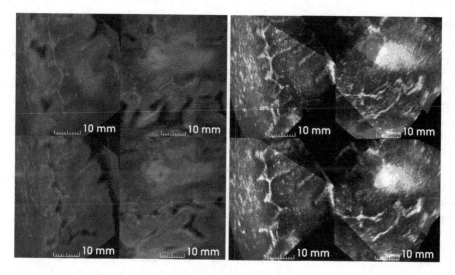

Fig. 3. Axial and sagittal views of the registration results in both tasks—MRI-iUS (left) and iUS-iUS (right)—for case 27. The top row is the initial alignment, the bottom row after registration. The MR FLAIR image is depicted in grey scale, the pre-resection iUS image in magenta, and the post-resection iUS image in green. (Color figure online)

4   Discussion

In the two registration tasks of the CuRIOUS 2019 challenge, we observe a directional bias of the results, i.e. one direction outperforms the other one. As a consequence the symmetric approach which combines both directions underperforms. At the same time, the symmetric approach has the lowest standard deviation for the MR-iUS task and has a lower maximum TRE, i.e. the worst case is handled better.

One challenge of the multi-modal registration task is that iUS and MR images have fundamentally different image characteristics: voxel shape and size as well as the field of view are very different. Furthermore, the iUS images are affected by speckles and appear quite noisy. Those factors could explain the performance difference of the directional approaches. On the other hand, the mono-modal registration task shows similar directional bias. Here, the challenge lies in the tissue resection. In the pre-resection image, the tumour tissue is visible, but it has no correspondence in the post-resection image. When the pre-resection image is used as reference, blocks of the post-resection image with high variance are matched to it. The borders of the resected tissue are quite distinct in the post-resection images and are likely chosen for the block-matching. Those blocks do not have a correspondence in the pre-resection image and can thus impair the overall transformation estimation. This conclusion suggests that similar effects could take place in the mono-modal setting as well. Trying to finding correspondences of US speckles in the MR image will most likely not provide a constructive match. The MR image is less noisy with clearer structures and is thus more suitable to determine the blocks to be matched. Noise reduction, specifically speckle reduction in the ultrasound images might reduce those effects. Different similarity measures than the used NCC might also improve the registration further. Improving the discrepancy between the directional approaches could yield an even better symmetric result whose advantages are currently held back by the bad performance of one directional registration in both tasks. The initial landmark distance is 5.37 mm for the MR-iUS task and 3.55 mm for the

Table 1. Mean TRE in mm per case for the MR-iUS registration task evaluated on all cases with landmark pairs provided for this task. The chosen setting is: reference US, affine, $ln = 2$, and $v = 25$.

Case	Initial	Rigid	Affine	Oracle
1	1.82	1.70	1.72	1.07
2	5.68	5.32	2.90	1.13
3	9.58	3.40	1.48	0.77
4	2.99	1.52	1.56	0.98
5	12.02	9.90	3.47	0.94
6	3.27	1.87	1.87	0.78
7	1.82	1.42	2.45	1.26
8	2.63	2.51	2.59	1.08
12	19.68	19.16	16.37	0.94
13	4.57	3.54	2.18	0.96
14	3.03	1.50	2.11	1.00
15	3.21	2.39	2.46	1.30
16	3.39	1.95	1.61	0.91
17	6.39	1.90	2.11	1.04
18	3.56	1.28	1.45	0.76
19	3.28	2.22	2.99	0.83
21	4.55	1.78	2.00	0.75
23	7.01	4.04	1.66	0.71
24	1.10	1.63	1.32	0.75
25	10.06	6.91	1.34	0.90
26	2.83	1.33	1.50	0.98
27	5.76	2.09	1.80	1.03
mean	**5.37**	**3.61**	**2.68**	**0.95**
stddev	**4.17**	**3.97**	**3.04**	**0.16**

Table 2. Mean TRE in mm per case for the iUS-iUS registration task evaluated on all cases with landmark pairs provided for this task. The chosen setting is: reference US-after, rigid, $ln = 2$, and $v = 25$.

Case	Initial	Rigid	Affine	Oracle
1	5.80	1.34	2.04	0.97
2	3.65	4.63	5.44	1.62
3	2.91	1.34	7.81	0.68
4	2.22	0.91	2.13	0.56
6	2.12	3.07	4.06	1.25
7	3.62	2.61	3.20	1.47
12	3.97	1.65	1.63	1.10
14	0.63	0.60	0.61	0.45
15	1.63	0.90	0.87	0.72
16	3.13	3.12	2.87	1.09
17	5.71	1.83	2.29	0.97
18	5.29	2.29	2.32	1.16
19	2.05	1.81	3.90	0.89
21	3.35	1.87	1.20	0.81
24	2.61	1.06	1.93	0.64
25	7.61	2.84	5.76	0.92
27	3.98	0.71	0.62	0.47
mean	**3.55**	**1.92**	**2.86**	**0.93**
stddev	**1.70**	**1.04**	**1.93**	**0.32**

iUS-iUS task. Only a few cases have clearly higher mean distance and for these, two levels of the pyramidal approach have a sufficient capture range. Higher values of ln show little effect in the mono-modal task. For the multi-modal task, higher ln even worsen the alignment of many registration settings. If there are already difficulties in finding correct correspondences in the finer levels, coarser levels will not improve this. Increasing the percentage of matched blocks from 10% to 25% improves the mTRE over all settings. Increasing it further to match all floating image blocks does not show a clear advantage but increases the computational time. A value of 25% for v thus seems a good choice. Despite these limitations, overall good registration results can be achieved by using this registration framework with mostly default parameters. The initial average landmark distance of 5.37 mm and 3.55 mm was reduced to 2.68 mm and 1.92 mm for the MR-iUS and the iUS-iUS task respectively.

Acknowledgments. This work is supported by the UCL EPSRC Centre for Doctoral Training in Medical Imaging [EP/L016478/1], the Wellcome/EPSRC Centre for Interventional and Surgical Sciences [NS/A000050/1], the Wellcome/EPSRC Centre for Medical Engineering [WT 203148/Z/16/Z] and EPSRC [NS/A000027/1]. We gratefully acknowledge the support of NVIDIA Corporation with the donation of the Quadro P6000 used for this research. This research was supported by the NIHR BRC based at GSTT and KCL.

References

1. Drobny, D., Vercauteren, T., Ourselin, S., Modat, M.: Registration of MRI and iUS data to compensate brain shift using a symmetric block-matching based approach. In: Stoyanov, D., et al. (eds.) POCUS/BIVPCS/CuRIOUS/CPM -2018. LNCS, vol. 11042, pp. 172–178. Springer, Cham (2018). https://doi.org/10.1007/978-3-030-01045-4_21
2. Ebner, M., et al.: Volumetric reconstruction from printed films: enabling 30 year longitudinal analysis in MR neuroimaging. NeuroImage **165**, 238–250 (2018)
3. Markiewicz, P.J., et al.: NiftyPET: a high-throughput software platform for high quantitative accuracy and precision PET imaging and analysis. Neuroinformatics **16**(1), 95–115 (2017)
4. Modat, M., Cash, D.M., Daga, P., Winston, G.P., Duncan, J.S., Ourselin, S.: Global image registration using a symmetric block-matching approach. J. Med. Imaging (Bellingham) **1**(2), 024003 (2014)
5. Niftyreg github page. https://github.com/KCL-BMEIS/niftyreg/wiki. Accessed 29 July 2019
6. Ourselin, S., Roche, A., Subsol, G., Pennec, X., Ayache, N.: Reconstructing a 3D structure from serial histological sections. Image Vis. Comput. **19**(1–2), 25–31 (2001)
7. Xiao, Y., et al.: Evaluation of MRI to ultrasound registration methods for brain shiftcorrection: the CuRIOUS2018 challenge. IEEE Trans. Med. Imaging (2019). https://doi.org/10.1109/TMI.2019.2935060

8. Xiao, Y., Fortin, M., Unsgård, G., Rivaz, H., Reinertsen, I.: REtroSpective evaluation of cerebral tumors (RESECT): a clinical database of pre-operative MRI and intra-operative ultrasound in low-grade glioma surgeries. Med. Phys. **44**(7), 3875–3882 (2017)
9. Yushkevich, P.A., Avants, B.B., Das, S.R., Pluta, J., Altinay, M., Craige, C.: Bias in estimation of hippocampal atrophy using deformation-based morphometry arises from asymmetric global normalization: an illustration in ADNI 3T MRI data. NeuroImage **50**(2), 434–445 (2010)

Comparing Deep Learning Strategies and Attention Mechanisms of Discrete Registration for Multimodal Image-Guided Interventions

In Young Ha$^{(\boxtimes)}$ ⓘ and Mattias P. Heinrich ⓘ

University of Luebeck, Ratzeburger Allee 160, Luebeck, Germany
{ha,heinrich}@imi.uni-luebeck.de

Abstract. In medical imaging, deep learning has been applied to segmentation and classification tasks successfully, whereas its use for image
registration tasks is still limited. The use of discrete registration can
alleviate the problems limiting the use of CNN based registration for
large displacements by helping to capture more complex deformations.
We evaluate different building blocks of learning based discrete registration for the CuRIOUS multimodal image registration challenge. We also
propose a new attention module, which estimates information contents of
a grid point, compare different loss functions and evaluate the influence
of self-supervised pre-training of feature extraction step.

Keywords: Deep learning · Discrete registration · Multimodal
registration · CuRIOUS challenge

1 Introduction and Related Work

The CuRIOUS challenge evaluates algorithms for the multimodal registration of
intra-operative ultrasound scans to pre-operative MRI diagnostic scans to guide
image-based interventions of tumour resection [9]. While deep learning has been
successfully applied to many segmentation and classification tasks in medical
imaging, its use for image registration appears to be more challenging. This is
evident in the first challenge in 2018, where only few deep learning based method
participated, and the only one applied to the test dataset achieved comparatively
poor results [9]. Yet the use of deep convolutional networks in image-guided
interventions would be very relevant given their immense potential for speed-up
at inference time. The most recent work for learning based registration often
required both self-supervised and weakly-supervised cost functions and fairly
large annotated training datasets [1,7] to reach the accuracy of conventional
methods or still required many iterative steps [2]. In [5], we argue that the use
of discrete registration can alleviate the problems presently limiting the use of

This work is funded by the German Research Foundation DFG (HE 7364/2).

© Springer Nature Switzerland AG 2019
L. Zhou et al. (Eds.): LABELS 2019/HAL-MICCAI 2019/CuRIOUS 2019, LNCS 11851, pp. 145–151, 2019.
https://doi.org/10.1007/978-3-030-33642-4_16

CNN based registration for large displacements. The key insight is that using a discrete displacement search similar to classical block-matching can help to capture more complex deformations as also demonstrated in 2D optical flow estimation in [3], where this step without trainable weights was coined correlation layer. In discrete registration, a dense 3D displacement map is predicted for each control point of the fixed image that measures the dissimilarity for all potential deformations with respect to the moving image (in our case a map of size $11 \times 11 \times 11$ capturing a spatial region of $+-$ 20 voxels or 10 mm). Two important challenges specific to intra-operative ultrasound to MRI registration currently prevail:

(1) the definition of similarity and extraction of modality-invariant features is difficult,
(2) the large differences in field of view necessitate a strategy to detect potentially uninformative regions that may deteriorate the transformation and focus the attention to areas of good structural content.

1.1   Contributions

In this work, we compare the most relevant building blocks of learning based discrete registration and propose a number of new strategies that deal with the above mentioned challenges. First, we introduce a new attention module that estimates the information content of a grid point based on its spatial displacement map. Second, we compare different loss functions, including CNN-based heatmaps, for the definition of errors in predicted displacement maps used for backpropagation. Third, we evaluate the influence of self-supervised pre-training of the feature extraction step based on hand-crafted self-similarity context descriptors [6].

2   Methods

Our method builds upon the discrete block-matching strategy presented in [4]. In this work we, however, restrict ourselves to a one-step single-level registration (yet an extension would likely yield more accurate results). The general overview of our method is shown in Figs. 1 and 2. First, a feature network is used to extract slightly downsampled 24-channel representations of the original input images (that have been resampled to 0.5 mm isotropic resolution). 2. Second, a 3D displacement map of size $11 \times 11 \times 11$ is computed for a number of coarse control points on a regular grid using the sum of squared difference metric of the extracted features (similar to [3] and [5]). 3. Third, the final (regularised) displacement probabilities and thus the correspondences are obtained either by directly applying a softmax operator to the negative scaled dissimilarity values or using another small CNN network that works on the displacement dimensions. Optionally, an attention weight is computed for each grid location to discard or down-weigh unreliable correspondences. Finally, a least squares regression is used to compute a rigid or affine transformation based to the found correspondences. The individual steps are explained in more detail in Table 1.

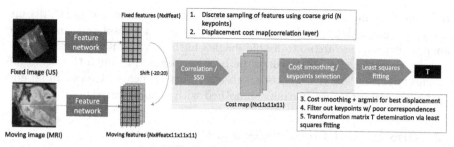

Fig. 1. An Overview of the proposed framework with learned features (feature network in Table 2). (The baseline method uses a handcrafted MIND-SSC descriptor for feature extraction.) The part with gray background can be replaced with a convolutional network, which learns the attention weights (see Fig. 2).

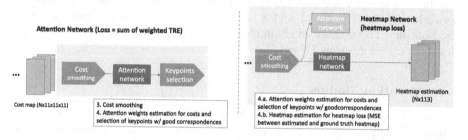

Fig. 2. An Overview of the proposed frameworks, which use attention network (left) and heatmap loss (right). For the heatmap loss ground truth heatmaps are generated based on the landmark coordinates.

2.1 Feature Network

We compare the use of fixed handcrafted MIND-SSC self-similarity context descriptors [6] to a trainable CNN network to extract modality-invariant representations. The networks weights are shared between MRI and US and the network architecture consists of the blocks as described in Table 1.

Since our initial tests indicated that learning these features from scratch could be challenging due to the limited supervision and strong appearance differences, we also conducted experiments in which a self-supervised learning of CNN features with a mean-squared error (MSE) loss against the handcrafted SSC features (12 channels each for 4 neighbouring locations = 48 features per voxel).

2.2 3D Dense Displacement (correlation) Layer

Next, a 3D displacement map of size $11 \times 11 \times 11$ is computed for a number of coarse control points on a regular grid (every seventh voxel in all 3 dimensions) using the SSD metric of the 48-dimensional features that measures the dissimilarity between a fixed location in the fixed image and a displaced voxel in the moving image. There are no trainable weights in this layer, but in order to reduce memory overhead (the loss needs to be back propagated through this layer) we use checkpointing and a loop over a subset of displacements. As done in [4] and [5] the dissimilarities are spatially smoothed with a small kernel.

2.3 Displacement Probabilities and Correspondences

To convert the dissimilarity maps into displacement probabilities the FlowNet approach used a very parameter-intensive fully-connected architecture for the respective channels (441 in their case of a 21×21 displacement map). We argue that a 3D convolutional network is much more appropriate and can substantially reduce the number of required parameters and subsequently the necessary training dataset. The proposed network architecture is a fully-convolutional 3D network that takes a $1 \times 11 \times 11 \times 11$ Tensor as input and produces a same-sized output. The number of channels in kernel sizes of the network (Heatmap Network) are as given in Table 1.

2.4 Attention Module

In the conventional discrete registration of [4] a number of heuristics are employed to filter out unreliable correspondences. The 50th percentile of the minimum displacement map value is used to discard potentially poor matches. In addition a trimmed least squares optimisation is performed to filter out further correspondences that do not follow a rigid or affine transformation model. Here, we take inspiration of [8] and train an attention module that takes the $11 \times 11 \times 11$ displacement map as input and uses a small 3D convolutional network followed by a sigmoid to predict a scalar attention value. It consists of the blocks as described in Table 1 in our experiments.

3 Experiments

3.1 Loss Functions

We either use an MSE-Loss on the predicted displacement probabilities in comparison to ground truth heatmaps generated from the known correspondences in the training data (assuming a rigid transformation of the landmarks) or directly minimise the target registration error after least-squares fitting. The latter could have the disadvantage of losing gradient strength through many iterations of solving a linear system of equations, while the former requires the empirical setting of a suitable Gauss kernel to define ground truth heatmaps.

Table 1. Details of network architectures. For each convolutional layer, number of input/output channels (first/second argument), kernel size (k), padding (p), stride (s) and dilation (d) values are given. * indicates that a Normalization layer (for Feature Network InstanceNorm3d and for rest BatchNorm3d) and a ReLU Unit (ReLU for Feature Network, PReLU for the other networks) is followed after the convolutional layer.

Feature Network	Attention Network	Heatmap Network
Conv3d(1,16, k=5, p=4, d=2)*	Conv3d(1,16, k=5, s=1)*	Conv3d(1,8,k=3,p=1)*
Conv3d(16,32, k=3, s=1, p=1)*	Conv3d(16,16,k=3)*	Conv3d(8,16,k=3,s=2,p=1)*
Conv3d(32,64, k=3, s=1, p=1)*	Conv3d(16,16, k=3)*	Conv3d(16,32,k=1)*
Conv3d(64,48, k=3, s=1, p=1)	Conv3d(16,16,k=3)*	Upsample(size=(11,11,11))
Sigmoid()	Conv3d(16,1,k=1)	Conv3d(32,16,k=3,p=1)*
	Sigmoid()	Conv3d(16,8,k=3,p=1)*
		Conv3d(8,1,k=3,p=1)

3.2   Ablation Study

To determine the effectiveness of each module, we performed an ablation study based on different combination of the modules. For all experiments we use nine pairs from the CuRIOUS training dataset, case 1–9 and 12, learning rate of 0.005 and the networks are trained for 100 epochs.

As for the **baseline** framework, we use a hand-crafted MIND-SSC descriptor to extract features from the images. From the features we then determine control points using a coarse regular grid and compute the correlation of the fixed and moving patches within the 20 voxel range (displacement from -20 voxels to 20 voxels). The cost map obtained from the correlation layer is then smoothed and regularized (softmax), which is then multiplied with the displacement grid to obtain best displacement vectors for the control points. As mentioned in Sect. 2.4, only the 50th percentile of the minimum displacement map values is used to select control points with good correspondences. The selected control points are then given as input to a trimmed least square optimization function, from which we obtain a transformation matrix. From this baseline framework, we substitute the MIND-SSC descriptor with a pre-trained feature network, which is trained weakly-supervised based on the TRE loss. The **feature network** (Sect. 2.1) shows comparable results as the baseline method, while being slightly faster.

The goal of the **attention network** is to filter out unreliable correspondences by assigning appropriate weights to the control points with poor correspondences. For the training of this network, the sum of weighted TRE is used.

In addition to different networks, the framework is also trained using different loss functions, where we use a heatmap instead of directly comparing the distance between landmarks. A ground truth heatmap is required for this part and it can be generated as described in Sect. 2.3. Based on the output of this **heatmap network**, the best displacement vectors are determined and using attention module, control points with poor correspondences are filtered out before computing a transformation between landmark vectors of US and MRI images.

Finally, we train the feature network and the attention network simultaneously (**end-to-end**), with the feature network initialized with good weights (**fine-tuning**) and random initialization (**from scratch**).

4 Results and Discussion

The result of the experiments are presented in Table 2. Although the feature network can simulate the MIND descriptor sufficiently and reach similar result as baseline method, learning attention weights for optimal cost seems to be difficult, especially when large displacement values are present. The use of heatmap loss led to poor result in our experiment setting and took longer to compute. The possible reason for this result can be the sub-optimal selection of the size of the Gauss Kernel.

The end-to-end training of feature network and attention network was performed in two different variations; with a good initialization and with a random initialization. As expected, the network reaches better accuracy when initialized with a good weights.

Table 2. Quantitative comparative evaluation of CuRIOUS dataset (TREs in mm). We demonstrate advantages of (1) using learned features vs. handcrafted self-similarity MIND-SSC descriptors, (2) using attention module, (3) computing loss based on the ground truth heatmap vs based on target registration error after least-squares fitting.

Method	(1)	(2)	(3)	2	5	7	13	17	23	Mean	Duration
No registration				5.75	12.20	1.88	4.71	6.41	7.05	5.29	–
Baseline	✗	✗	✗	3.62	2.49	2.27	1.67	1.62	1.37	2.35	0.33 s
Feat-net	✔	✗	✗	3.80	2.40	2.44	1.78	1.79	1.33	2.50	0.24 s
Attention-net	✗	✔	✗	6.08	14.19	2.58	3.60	5.42	2.11	4.50	0.35 s
Feat + Attention-net	✔	✔	✗	5.45	12.77	2.52	4.47	4.36	2.07	4.30	0.25 s
Heatmap loss	✗	✔	✔	5.82	11.67	3.85	3.50	4.77	4.32	5.11	0.61 s
End-to-end (fine-tuning)	✔	✔	✗	4.38	9.07	3.24	6.62	4.33	4.64	4.47	0.25 s
End-to-end (from scratch)	✔	✔	✗	4.36	8.06	4.06	6.93	7.04	5.36	5.02	0.25 s

5 Outlook

In this paper, we have presented a comparison between different building blocks of learning based discrete registration. Learned features are as good as handcrafted features, whereas the learned attention weights for out-filtering poor correspondence keypoints does not seem to work as we expected. As future work, we plan to perform further experiments, which include optimisation of hyperparameters, use of augmentation, multi-level registration and estimation of symmetric transformation.

References

1. Balakrishnan, G., Zhao, A., Sabuncu, M.R., Guttag, J., Dalca, A.V.: VoxelMorph: a learning framework for deformable medical image registration. IEEE Trans. Med. Imaging **38**(8), 1788–1800 (2019)
2. Blendowski, M., Heinrich, M.P.: Learning interpretable multi-modal features for alignment with supervised iterative descent. In: International Conference on Medical Imaging with Deep Learning, pp. 73–83 (2019)
3. Dosovitskiy, A., et al.: FlowNet: learning optical flow with convolutional networks. In: Proceedings of the IEEE International Conference on Computer Vision, pp. 2758–2766 (2015)
4. Heinrich, M.P.: Intra-operative ultrasound to MRI fusion with a public multimodal discrete registration tool. In: Stoyanov, D., et al. (eds.) POCUS/BIVPCS/CuRIOUS/CPM 2018. LNCS, vol. 11042, pp. 159–164. Springer, Cham (2018). https://doi.org/10.1007/978-3-030-01045-4_19
5. Heinrich, M.P.: Closing the gap between deep and conventional image registration using probabilistic dense displacement networks. In: Shen, D., et al. (eds.) MICCAI 2019, Part VI. LNCS, vol. 11769, pp. 50–58. Springer, Cham (2019). https://doi.org/10.1007/978-3-030-32226-7_6
6. Heinrich, M.P., Jenkinson, M., Papież, B.W., Brady, S.M., Schnabel, J.A.: Towards realtime multimodal fusion for image-guided interventions using self-similarities. In: Mori, K., Sakuma, I., Sato, Y., Barillot, C., Navab, N. (eds.) MICCAI 2013, Part I. LNCS, vol. 8149, pp. 187–194. Springer, Heidelberg (2013). https://doi.org/10.1007/978-3-642-40811-3_24
7. Hering, A., Kuckertz, S., Heldmann, S., Heinrich, M.P.: Enhancing label-driven deep deformable image registration with local distance metrics for state-of-the-art cardiac motion tracking. In: Handels, H., Deserno, T., Maier, A., Maier-Hein, K., Palm, C., Tolxdorff, T. (eds.) Bildverarbeitung für die Medizin 2019. Informatik aktuell, pp. 309–314. Springer, Wiesbaden (2019). https://doi.org/10.1007/978-3-658-25326-4_69
8. Schlemper, J., et al.: Attention gated networks: learning to leverage salient regions in medical images. Med. Image Anal. **53**, 197–207 (2019)
9. Xiao, Y., et al.: Evaluation of MRI to ultrasound registration methods for brain shift correction: The curious2018 challenge. arXiv preprint: arXiv:1904.10535 (2019)

Author Index

Printed in the United States
by Baker & Taylor Publisher Services